COVID-19, Neuroimmunology and Neural Function

Edited by Thomas Heinbockel and Robert Weissert

Published in London, United Kingdom

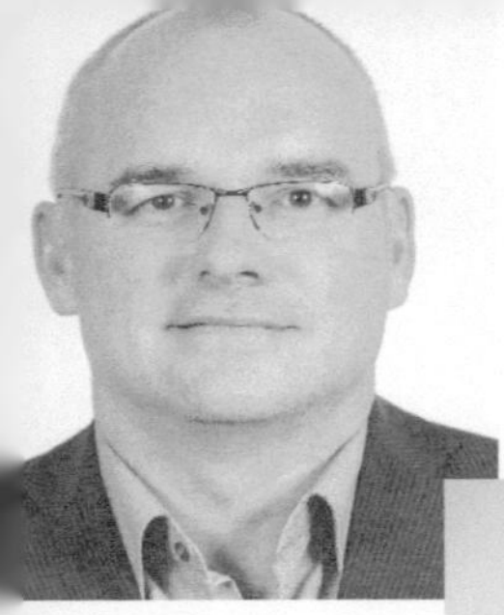
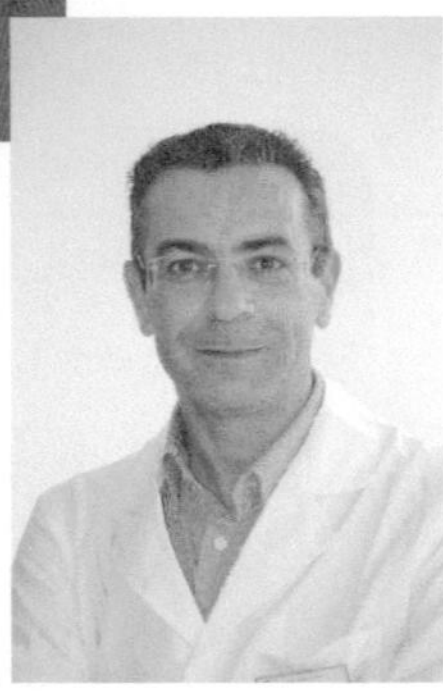
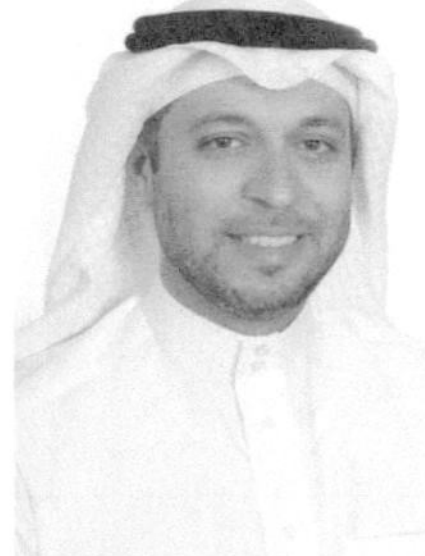
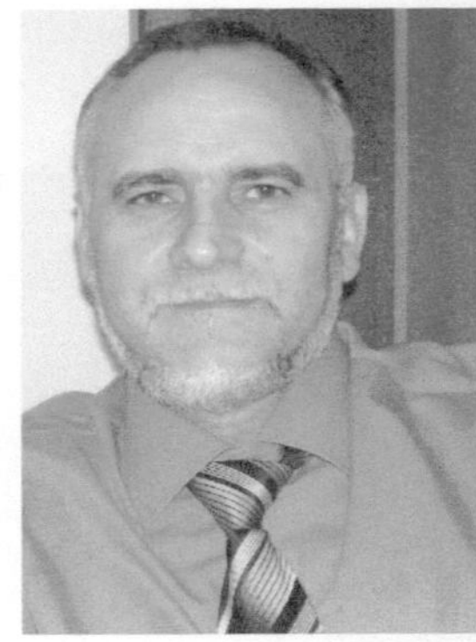
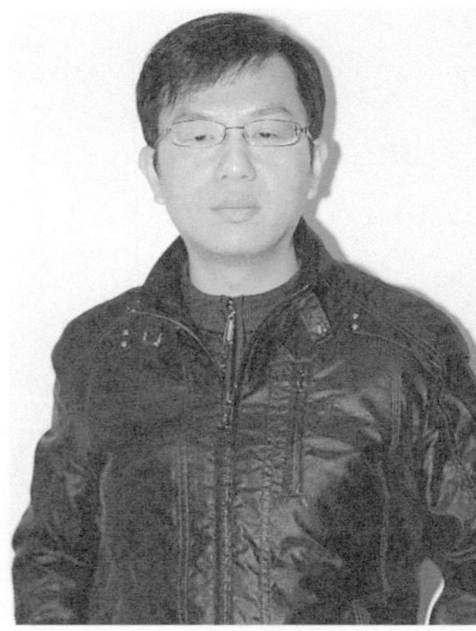
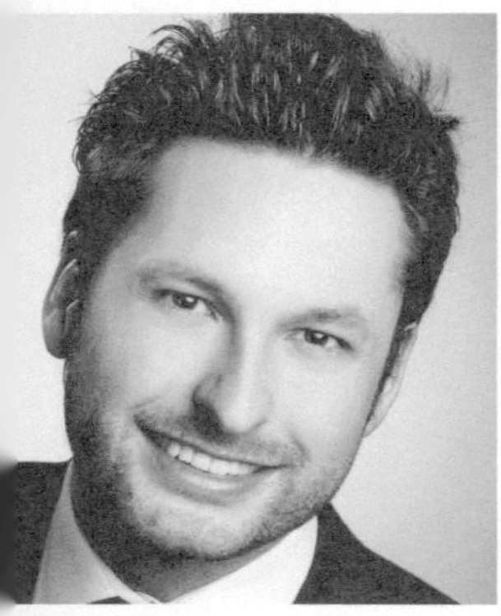
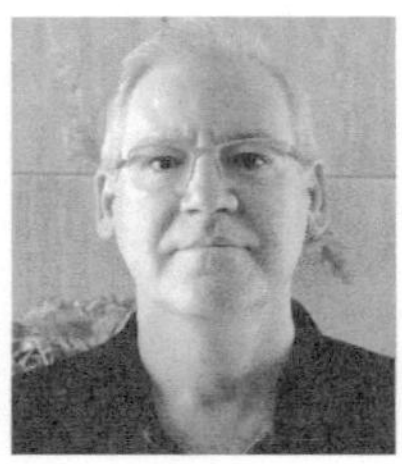

IntechOpen

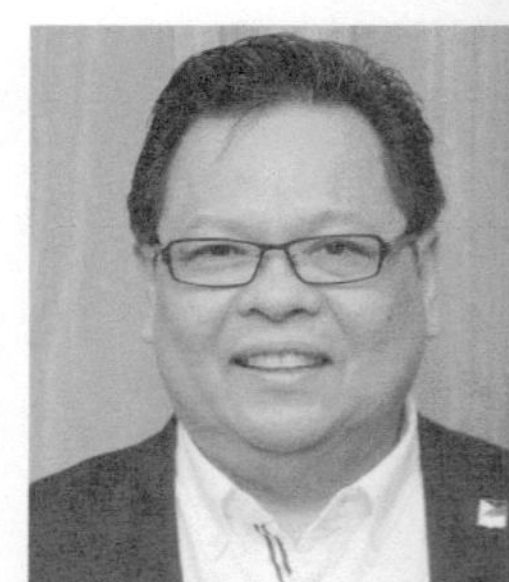
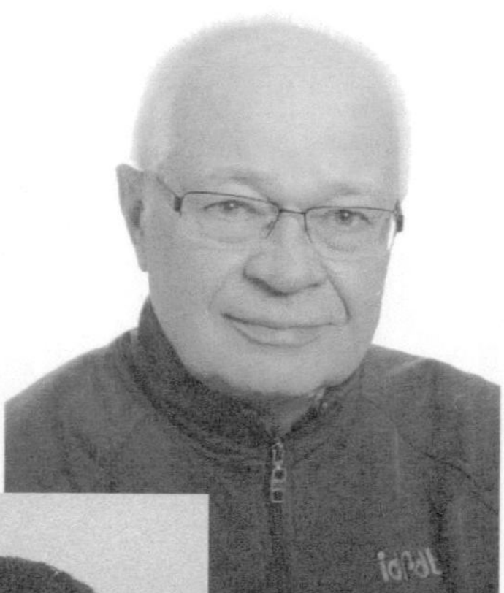
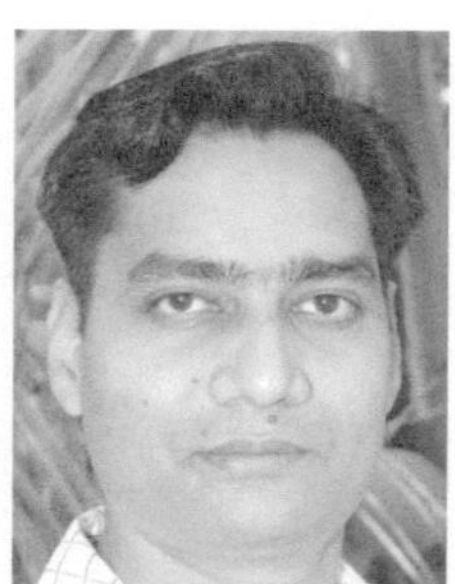
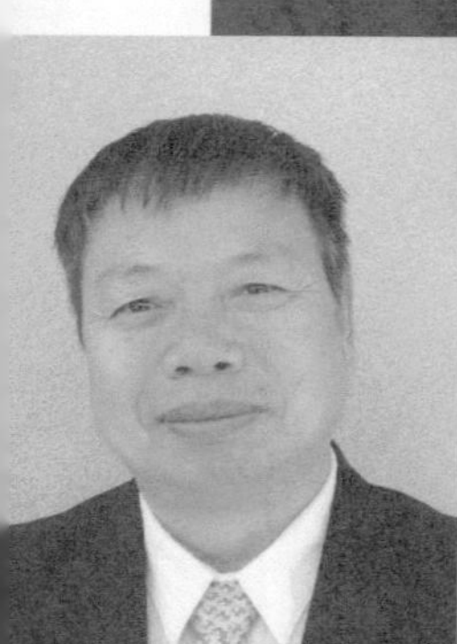
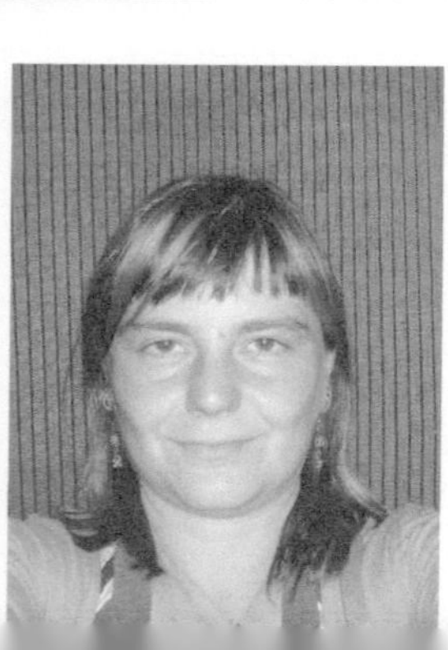
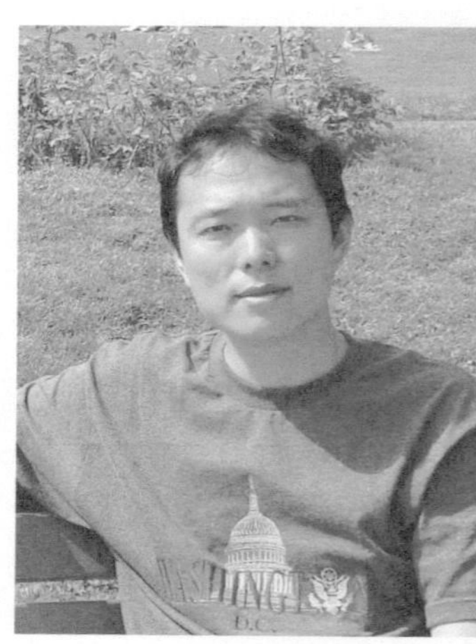

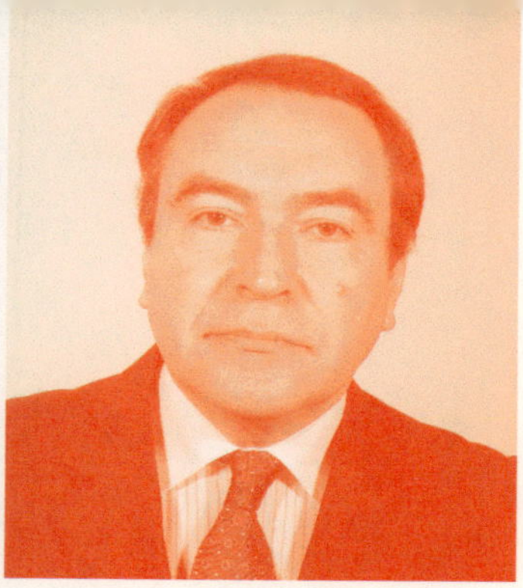

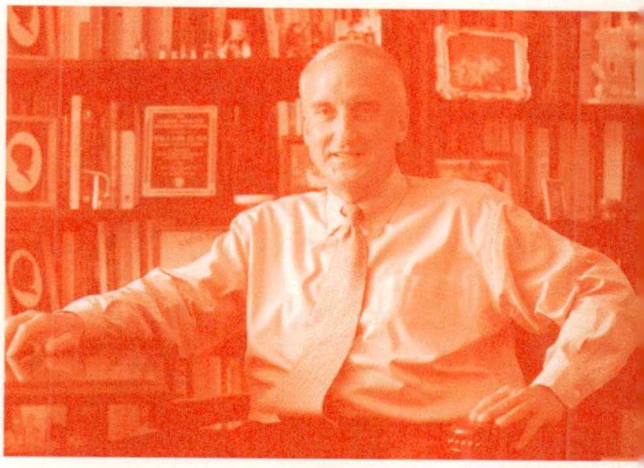

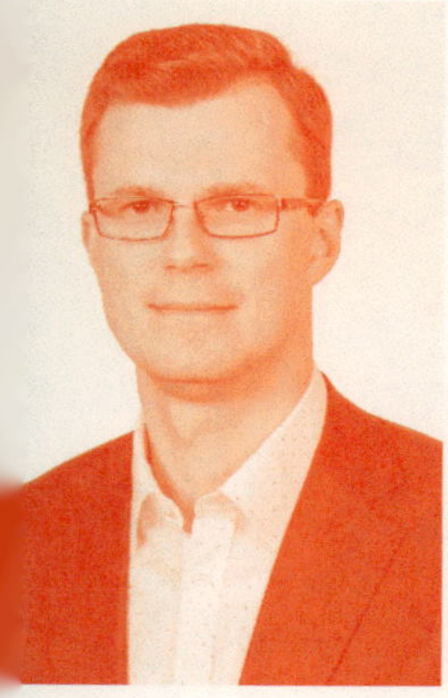

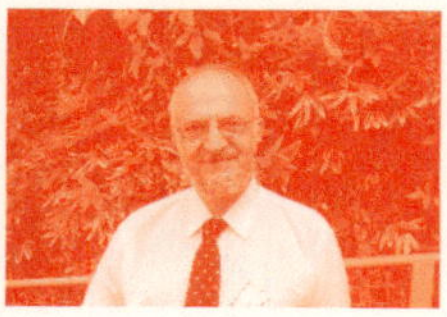

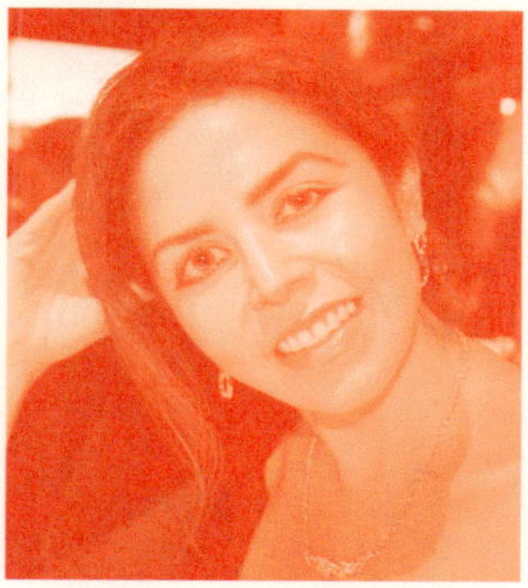

Supporting open minds since 2005

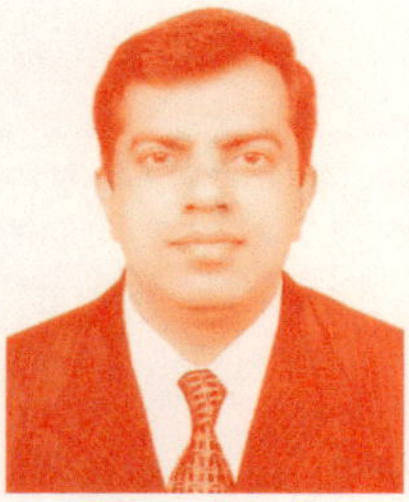

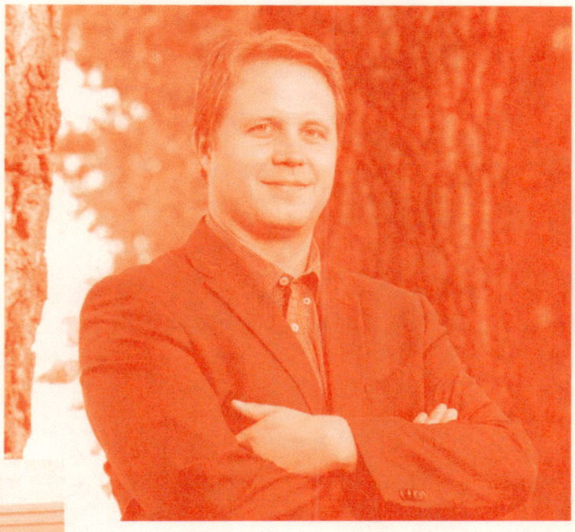

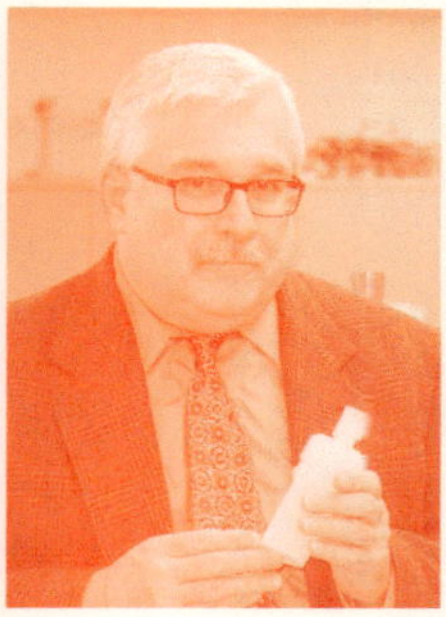

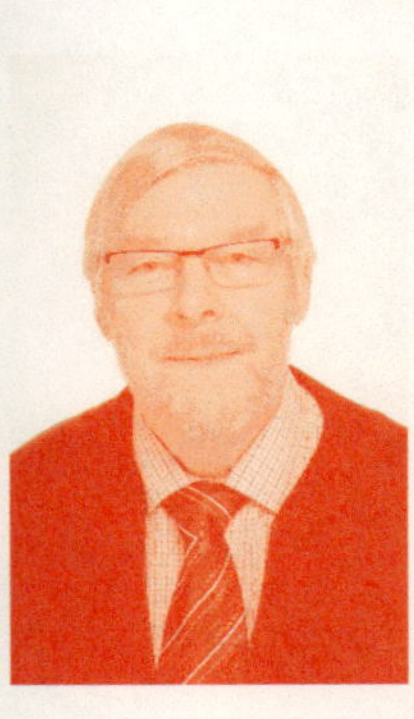

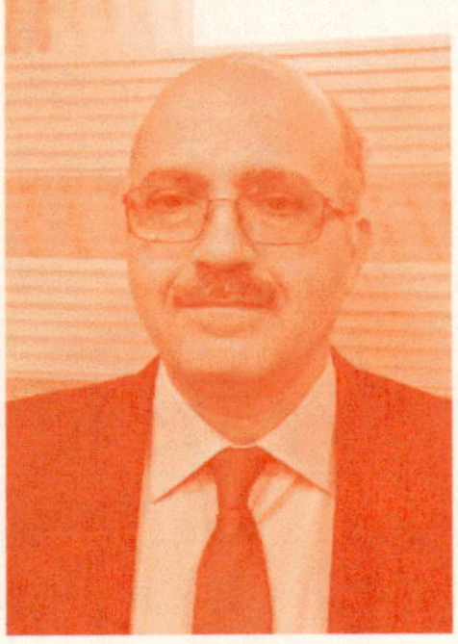

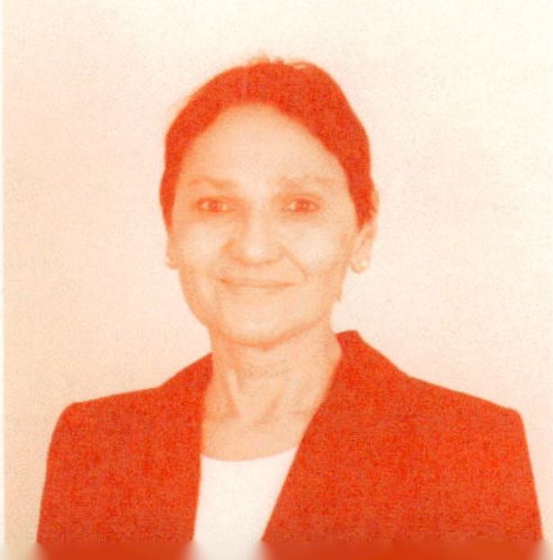

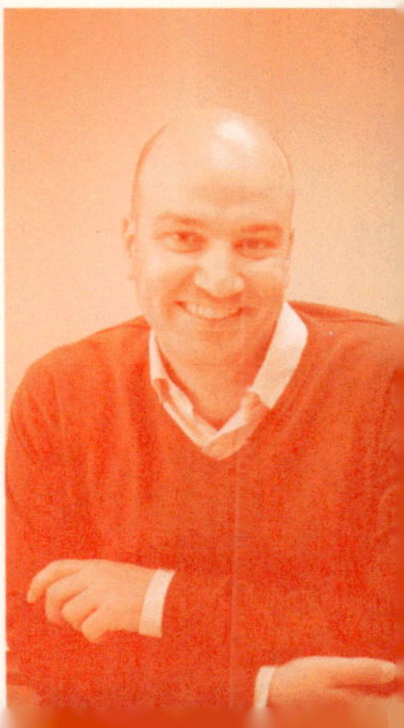

COVID-19, Neuroimmunology and Neural Function
http://dx.doi.org/10.5772/intechopen.95199
Edited by Thomas Heinbockel and Robert Weissert

Contributors
Andreia Monteiro, Artur Paiva, Ana Mafalda Fonseca, Robert Weissert, Saraswathi Ilango, Saikarthik Jayakumar, Abdul Rahman Al-Atram, Shona Pfeiffer, Steven G. Fagan, Pedro Guimarães, Rafael Jesus, Carolina Azoia, Paulo Coelho, Yaroslav R. Nartsissov

First published in London, United Kingdom, 2022 by IntechOpen
IntechOpen is the global imprint of INTECHOPEN LIMITED, registered in England and Wales, registration number: 11086078, 5 Princes Gate Court, London, SW7 2QJ, United Kingdom
Printed in Croatia

British Library Cataloguing-in-Publication Data
A catalogue record for this book is available from the British Library

Additional hard and PDF copies can be obtained from orders@intechopen.com

COVID-19, Neuroimmunology and Neural Function
Edited by Thomas Heinbockel and Robert Weissert
p. cm.
Print ISBN 978-1-80355-030-5
Online ISBN 978-1-80355-031-2
eBook (PDF) ISBN 978-1-80355-032-9

Meet the editors

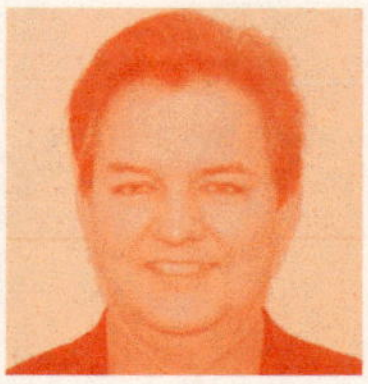

Thomas Heinbockel, Ph.D., is a professor and interim chair, Department of Anatomy, Howard University College of Medicine, Washington, DC. He holds an adjunct faculty position in both the Department of Anatomy & Neurobiology and the Department of Physiology, University of Maryland School of Medicine. Dr. Heinbockel studied biology at the Philipps-University, Germany. His studies of the brain started during his MS thesis work at the Max Planck Institute for Behavioral Physiology, Germany. Dr. Heinbockel earned a Ph.D. in Neuroscience at the University of Arizona, USA. After graduating, he worked as a research associate at the Institute of Physiology, Otto-von-Guericke University, Germany. Dr. Heinbockel's research is focused on understanding how the brain processes information as it relates to neurological and psychiatric disorders. His laboratory at Howard University concentrates on foundational and translational topics such as drug development, organization of the olfactory and limbic systems, and neural signaling and synaptic transmission in the central nervous system.

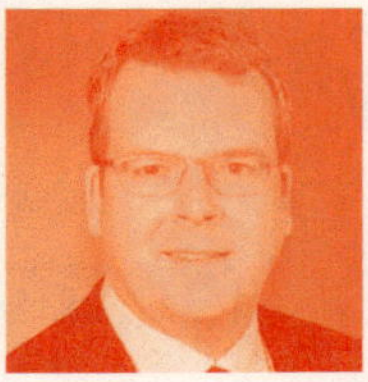

Robert Weissert, MD, Ph.D., did his training in neurology, neuroimmunology, immunology, and genetics in Tuebingen, Germany; Miami and Chicago, USA; and the Karolinska Institute, Sweden. Between 1999 and 2007, in addition to his clinical duties as a neurologist at the University Hospital in Tuebingen, he headed a group of experimental neuroimmunology funded by the German Research Foundation (DFG) at the Hertie Institute of Clinical Brain Research. From 2007 to 2010, he worked as a director of research and development of a large pharmaceutical company in Geneva, Switzerland, and was a senior physician in the Department of Neurology, Cantonal Hospital, University of Geneva. Since 2011, Dr. Weissert has been working as a senior physician (neurology) and researcher at the University of Regensburg, Germany, where he had been a university professor of clinical neurobiology with a focus on neuroimmunology and neuroinflammation from 2012 to 2018. Since 2018, he has been an honorary professor at the University of Regensburg. Dr. Weissert has made important contributions to the understanding of the pathogenesis of neuroimmunological diseases and the establishment of novel treatment options with a focus on multiple sclerosis.

Contents

Preface

The recent and ongoing COVID-19 pandemic has changed societies and research around the world. As a result, this new book reflects the latest developments in the field of neuroscience related to these changes. It includes six chapters over two sections: "COVID-19 Effects: Neurology, Neuroimmunology, Neurogenesis" and "Molecular and Cellular Neurochemistry." The book presents comprehensive reviews in these different areas written by experts in their respective fields. COVID-19 is featured prominently and is a recurring theme throughout most chapters.

Neuroscience itself is a flourishing academic field that contributes to our understanding of molecular, cellular, and medical neurobiology. As scientific disciplines, neurobiology and neurochemistry study the role of chemicals that build the nervous system, explore the function of neurons and glial cells in health and disease, discover aspects of cell metabolism and neurotransmission, and reveal how degenerative processes are at work in the nervous system. This book is a valuable resource for neurobiologists, neurochemists, and other scientists alike. In addition, it will contribute to the training of current and future neuroscientists and, hopefully, will lead us on the path to curing some of the biggest challenges in human health.

Section 1 begins with Chapter 1, "Does COVID-19 Affect Adult Neurogenesis? A Neurochemical Perspective" by Jayakumar Saikarthik, Ilango Saraswathi and Abdulrahman A. Al-Atram. The chapter begins with a discussion of the impact of COVID-19 on adult neurogenesis with an emphasis on the role of ACE2 and neurotransmitters.

Chapter 2, "Neuroimmunology and Neurological Manifestations of COVID-19" by Robert Weissert, provides a comprehensive review of the neurological symptoms resulting from COVID-19 as it affects the nervous system, in addition to the respiratory symptoms due to an attack of the broncho-alveolar system. The chapter also addresses vaccination and therapeutic approaches to prevent COVID-19 effects on the nervous system.

Chapter 3, "COVID-19 and Seizures" by Rafael Jesus, Carolina Azoia, Paulo Coelho and Pedro Guimarães, reviews the association between COVID-19 and the mechanisms of acute symptomatic seizures through neurotropism and neuroinvasion features of SARS-CoV-2. The chapter reviews a variety of clinical presentations in this regard.

Section 2 begins with Chapter 4, "Peripheral Biomarkers in Multiple Sclerosis Patients Treated with Interferon-Beta," by Andreia Monteiro, Ana Mafalda Fonseca and Artur Paiva. It examines findings described in the literature that correlate specific alterations of different leukocytes subpopulations in the blood with disease status in multiple sclerosis patients. The authors argue that these have the potential to constitute a peripheral biomarker of disease progression.

Chapter 5, "Amino Acids as Neurotransmitters. The Balance between Excitation and Inhibition as a Background for Future Clinical Applications" by Yaroslav R. Nartissov, reviews the role of the neurotransmitters glycine and glutamate. The author proposes that, in addition to their obvious effects on the brain, their potential role in therapeutic treatment of pathological conditions needs to be explored.

Chapter 6, "Emerging Roles of Non-Coding RNA in Neuronal Function and Dysfunction" by Steven G. Fagan and Shona Pfeiffer, contributes a discussion of advancements in RNA sequencing technologies. The focus of the chapter is on the dysregulation, functions, and regulatory roles of novel small non-coding RNAs in the pathophysiological mechanisms of neurological disorders and their relevance as novel biomarkers of injury and therapeutic agents.

We are grateful to IntechOpen for initiating this book project and for asking us to serve as its editors. Many thanks go to Nera Butigan at IntechOpen for guiding us through the publication process and for moving the book ahead in a timely fashion. Thanks are due to all contributors to this book for their excellent chapters. Hopefully, all contributors will continue their research with many intellectual challenges and exciting new directions.

Thomas Heinbockel, Ph.D.
Professor and Interim Chair,
Department of Anatomy,
Howard University College of Medicine,
Washington, DC, USA

Robert Weissert, M.D. Ph.D.
Honorary Professor,
Attending in Neurology,
Department of Neurology,
University of Regensburg Hospital,
Regensburg, Germany

Section 1

COVID-19 Effects: Neurology, Neuroimmunology, Neurogenesis

Chapter 1

Does COVID-19 Affect Adult Neurogenesis? A Neurochemical Perspective

Jayakumar Saikarthik, Ilango Saraswathi and Abdulrahman A. Al-Atram

Abstract

COVID-19 has been found to cause neuropsychiatric symptoms which indicate brain involvement. SARS-CoV-2 may enter the brain by damaging and penetrating olfactory mucosa and via other possible routes like damaged blood–brain barrier, and hematologic spread. With SARS-CoV-2 having a higher affinity to ACE2 receptors, brain regions that have higher ACE2 receptors like the hippocampus, are more vulnerable to the effect of the viral invasion. In addition, immune cell activation, an important feature of COVID-19, leads to cytokine storm which causes neurotoxicity, neuroinflammation, and neurodegeneration. Impaired adult neurogenesis is related to many psychiatric disorders including depression, bipolar disorder, anxiety disorder, schizophrenia, and PTSD. It is known to be related to the depletion of neurotransmitters, dopamine, serotonin, norepinephrine, GABA, and glutamate which play a major role in adult neurogenesis. A recent study reveals that SSRI which acts by increasing serotonin is proven beneficial in COVID-19 patients. Thus, the current chapter will discuss the impact of COVID-19 on adult neurogenesis with emphasis on the role of ACE2 and neurotransmitters.

Keywords: COVID-19, SARS-CoV-2, ACE2, adult neurogenesis, glutamate, monoaminergic neurotransmitters, GABA

1. Introduction

The last two decades have seen epidemic outbreaks by novel viruses including SARS, MERS, and influenza which shared certain commonalities such as a likely zoonotic origin, high mortality rates, and less available therapeutic methods to counteract them. The COVID-19 pandemic shows no signs of slowing down with affecting 223 countries, with 224,811,910 cases, and 4,633,797 death tolls till date [1]. With what history on earlier pandemics has made us understand and with the rapidly mutating nature of the SARS-CoV-2 virus, it is not unreasonable to say that the pandemic is here to stay, and the world must learn to co-exist with it. The first reported case of COVID-19 was found in Wuhan, China in December 2019. By March 2020, the disease had spread across the globe and had become a public health emergency. The WHO declared a pandemic state to the disease spread on March 11, 2020 [2]. With more than a year since the declaration of the pandemic, the scientific community has yet not developed a definitive anti-viral drug to combat the disease spread. Even though the advent of vaccination has set the pace in favour of global health, we have a long way to go to eradicate if at all suppress the disease spread.

SARS-CoV-2 is highly virulent and highly contagious with the R0 value of 3.77 [3]. Though it predominantly affects the respiratory system, other organ systems like the gastrointestinal system, heart, kidney, and central nervous system are also targeted by the virus. Fever, chills, cough, shortness of breath or breathing difficulty, sore throat, nasal congestion, diarrhoea, nausea, vomiting, generalised body aches are some of the common symptoms noted in patients infected with COVID-19 [4].

Neurological manifestations of COVID-19 include non-specific symptoms like headache, dizziness, fatigue, and myopathy and more specific symptoms like anosmia, ageusia, impaired consciousness, stroke, meningitis, acute transverse myelitis, and Guillian-Barre syndrome [5, 6]. More than one third of the individuals with COVID-19 were found to present with neurological symptoms [7, 8]. The presence of viral RNA in cerebrospinal fluid and the brain was observed in COVID-19 patients [9]. Preliminary *in vitro* studies have found that SARS-CoV-2 can replicate in neuronal cells [10]. A post-mortem study has found that 48% of the studied cases had human CoV RNA in the CNS that was detectable [11]. SARS-CoV-2 is found to exhibit organotropism for the nervous system and SARS-CoV and MERS-CoV which are closely related to SARS-CoV-2 have neuro-invasive potential. Hence, apart from the secondary impact on the brain as a result of systemic complications like coagulopathy and hypoxia, the direct effect of SARS-CoV-2 infection on the brain and spinal cord is plausible and is being thoroughly studied by researchers globally. The neuropsychiatric symptoms in COVID-19 could be attributed to a variety of factors apart from the direct effect of the virus on the brain like psychological distress due to social isolation, the novelty of the disease spread and pandemic, concerns about family and friends contracting the disease, social stigma, etc. [12]. This chapter will, however, focus on the direct effects of the SARS-CoV-2 virus on the brain which could be attributed to the pathophysiology of neuropsychiatric symptoms with a special focus on ACE2 and monoaminergic neurotransmitters.

2. SARS-CoV-2

Coronaviruses are the largest among RNA viruses. They have a crown-like spikes on their surface and hence the name. SARS-CoV-2 is the latest/seventh coronavirus to become pathogenic to humans. It belongs to the Coronaviridae family which includes four genera; α−, β−, γ−, and δ-CoV. Out of these human pathogens include HCoV- 229E, HCoV- NL63 [α − CoV] and OC43, and HKU1 [β − CoV] that in most cases cause mild self-limiting respiratory disease. γ − and δ-CoV strains mainly affect avian species [13]. SARS-CoV and MERS-CoV, causatives of SARS and MERS, are beta coronaviruses that caused up to 9.6% and 34.3% mortality rates which were responsible for earlier pandemics that resulted in a death toll of 812 and 866, respectively [14]. SARS-CoV-2 is more similar to SARS-CoV and MERS-CoV while being far more pathogenic and transmissible than the earlier known coronaviruses.

SARS-CoV-2 is a beta coronavirus that is positive-sense single-stranded RNA virus with 29–30 kb in size. It has four structural proteins and 16 non-structural proteins. Nucleocapsid protein [N], membrane protein [M], spike protein [S], and envelope protein [E] are the four structural proteins (**Figure 1**). The capsid of the genome is formed by N protein and the genome is further surrounded by an envelope that is made up of M, E, and S proteins. Like other coronaviruses, SARS-CoV-2 has enveloped with a crown-like spikes on its surface. It is the spike protein that is responsible for the variations in host specificity and tissue tropism of the different coronavirus. Spike protein is a type-I membrane glycoprotein and has two functional

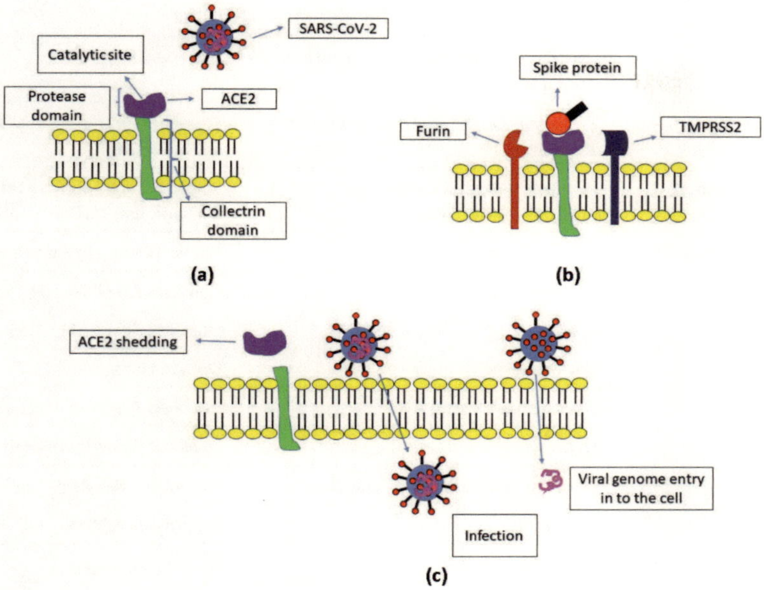

Figure 1.
(a) Structure of ACE2 and SARS-CoV-2; (b) Interaction of spike protein and ACE2; (c) Shedding of ACE2 and entry of SARS-CoV-2 into the cell.

subunits S1 and S2 with different functional domains in the amino and carboxy terminal. S1 subunit contains the receptor-binding domain [RBD] and binds with the receptor in the host cells. S2 subunit fuses the membranes of the host cells and the virus. The entry of the virus into the host cell involves binding of the S protein [S1 subunit] to a specific cell receptor followed by priming of the S protein by proteases in the host cell. This leads to the fusion of the spike protein to the cell membrane which is mediated by the S2 subunit [15]. The specific cell receptor through which SARS-CoV-2 enters the host cell is the ACE2 receptor and the protease in the host cell that processes the spike protein to reveal the fusion peptide between S1 and S2 subunits facilitating its entry, is a TMPRSS2 serine protease, member of the hepsin/TMPRSS subfamily [16]. Another protein named furin or paired basic amino acid cleaving enzyme [PACE], a member of the subtilisin-like proprotein convertase family, mediates proteolytic cut of the S protein at S1-S2 boundary, is required for TMPRSS2 processing of S protein. Both TMPRSS2 and furin are essential for the entry of SARS-CoV-2 into the cell. The furin cleavage site in the S protein of SARS-CoV-2 is not found in SARS-CoV and other beta coronaviruses [17].

3. ACE2

ACE2 is a cell surface protein, a metalloproteinase and an ectoenzyme which is an obligatory receptor for SARS-CoV and SARS-CoV-2. The affinity of SARS-CoV-2 to ACE2 is ten times higher than that of SARS-CoV which partly explains its higher pathogenicity [18]. It was discovered in 2000 by two independent groups of researchers while searching for human ACE homologues [19, 20]. The gene for ACE2 in humans is located in Xp22 and has 18 exons, a majority of which are similar to the exons of the ACE gene [21]. Despite ACE2 exhibiting 42% sequence identify and 61% sequence similarity with ACE, the two enzymes show enormous variations (**Table 1**) [27].

	ACE	ACE2
Forms	Exists as a 2-domain somatic form and a one domain testicular form	Exists as a single form
Structure	Transmembrane ectoenzyme with two active sites	Transmembrane ectoenzyme with one active site
Enzymatic action	Removes C-terminal dipeptide – peptidyl-dipeptidase	Removes single amino acid from C-terminus – carboxypeptidase
Substrate specificity	Converts Ang I to Ang II	Converts Ang I to Ang (1-9)
	Does not cleave Ang II	Converts Ang II to Ang (1-7)
	Converts Ang (1-9) to Ang (1-7)	Does not cleave Ang (1-9)
	Converts Ang (1-7) to Ang (1-5)	Does not cleave Ang (1-7)
	Does not cleave Ang A	Converts Ang A to Alamandine
	Hydrolyses bradykinin	Does not cleave bradykinin
	Does not cleave des-Arg9-bradykinin	Hydrolyses des-Arg9-bradykinin
Action on amyloid protein	Hydrolyses Aβ-43 to Aβ41	Hydrolyses Aβ43 to Aβ42
	Hydrolyses Aβ-42 to Aβ40	Does not cleave Aβ-42
Localisation within cells	Equal distribution between apical and basolateral membranes	Localised on the apical membrane
Transports intestinal amino acids	No	Transports intestinal neutral amino acids
Shedding into plasma	Unidentified. May involve metalloproteinase and A Disintegrin	By A Disintegrin and Metalloprotease 17 (ADAM 17)
Response to ACE inhibitor	Inhibited	Resistant, gets upregulated
Acts as a receptor to virus	No	Receptor for SARS-CoV and SARS-CoV-2

Table 1.
The comparison between ACE and ACE2 is given in **Table 1** *[22–26].*

Since the 20 years of its discovery, ACE2 was found to have a multitude of physiological and pathological functions based on its three fundamental actions viz. negative regulation of renin-angiotensin system [RAS], facilitation of amino acid transport in the intestine, and surface receptor for SARS-CoV and SARS-CoV-2. ACE2 is mainly expressed in the lungs, intestine, liver, heart, kidneys, testes, and brain. In the brain, it is expressed in neurons, astrocytes and oligodendrocytes, and in ventricles, substantia nigra, hypothalamus, hippocampus, middle temporal gyrus, posterior cingulate cortex, nuclei in pons—the nucleus of tractus solitarius and pre-Bötzinger complex and olfactory bulb [21, 28]. ACE2 expression is higher in astrocytes, astrocytic foot processes, pericytes, and endothelial cells which form the key components of the blood–brain barrier [29]. In the olfactory epithelium, its expression is higher in the supporting sustentacular cells than in olfactory sensory neurons [30]. The sites of ACE2 expression are given in **Table 2** [31].

3.1 Structure

ACE2 is a type 1 integral membrane protein that includes a short cytoplasmic C-terminus, a transmembrane region, collectrin, and N-terminal ectodomain. Zinc-binding motifs, HEMGH forms the active site of the enzyme. N-terminal domain

Vascular system	Endothelial cells, vascular smooth muscle cells, and migratory angiogenic cells
Heart	Cardiomyocytes, endothelial cells, pericytes, and epicardial adipose cells, and cardiofibroblasts
Skin	sebaceous gland cells and basal epidermal layer
Kidneys	glomerular endothelial cells, proximal tubule epithelial cells, bladder urothelial cells, luminal surface of tubular epithelial cells, and podocytes
Reproductive system	Ovary, oocyte, uterus, vagina, and placenta of the female reproductive system Adult Leydig cells and cells in the seminiferous ducts in the testis of the male reproductive system
Liver	Perinuclear hepatocytes, cholangiocytes, epithelial cells of the bile duct
Gut	Stratified epithelial cells of oesophagus, stomach, Intestinal epithelial cells, enterocytes of small intestine, absorptive enterocytes from the ileum, colon and rectum, and endothelial cells
Pancreas	Acinar cells and duct cells of the exocrine gland and alpha, beta, delta, and PP cells of islets of Langerhans
Thyroid	Glandular cells
Oral cavity	Tongue, buccal mucosa, gingiva, leucocytes within the oral mucosa, non-keratinising squamous epithelium of the oral cavity – basal layer
Upper airway	Ciliated epithelial cells, goblet cells
Lungs	Pulmonary vasculature, type I and II alveolar epithelial cells, bronchiolar epithelial cells
Eyes	Pigmented epithelial cells, photoreceptor cells, Müller glial cells
Central nervous system	Neurons, astrocytes, and oligodendrocytes, and in ventricles, substantia nigra, hypothalamus, hippocampus, middle temporal gyrus, posterior cingulate cortex, nuclei in pons – nucleus of tractus solitarius and pre-Bötzinger complex and olfactory bulb and cerebral vasculature and components of blood–brain barrier (astrocytes, astrocytic foot processes, pericytes, and endothelial cells)

Table 2.
Sites of ACE2 expression.

has a claw-shaped protease domain which is the binding site of receptor-binding domain [RBD] of SARS-CoV and SARS-CoV-2. N terminus is homologous to ACE and is a carboxypeptidase that metabolises peptides like angiotensin II, kinins, apelin-13, apelin-36, neurotensin 1–13, kinetensin, and morphins, and C terminus is homologous to collectrin which is involved in the trafficking of neutral amino acid transporter [B[o]AT1] in the intestinal epithelium [32].

4. Role of ACE2 in renin-angiotensin system [RAS]

Both ACE and ACE2 play a major role in maintaining renin-angiotensin system [RAS] homeostasis. ACE2 acts like a negative regulator of ACE in RAS. RAS involves a variety of proteins and enzymes. Angiotensinogen is an inactive precursor that gets cleaved by renin to form angiotensin I. ACE acts on angiotensin I to convert into angiotensin II [Ang II] while ACE2 converts Ang II to Ang [1-7]. Ang [1-7] then binds to Mas receptors and causes attenuation of the signal cascade that was activated by Ang II (**Figure 2**). Thus, ACE2 not only inactivates Ang II but also generates the antagonistic peptide Ang [1-7] [33]. Ang [1-7] can also be formed from Ang I by neutral endopeptidases and neprilysin, but the most effective pathway of Ang [1-7] generation is through ACE2 [34]. The conversion of Ang II

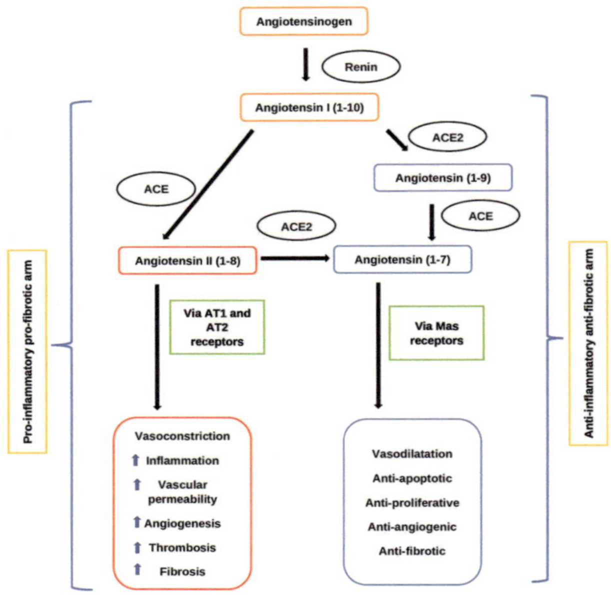

Figure 2.
Renin-Angiotensin System.

to Ang [1-7] by ACE2 is 70 folds more efficient than the conversion of Ang I to Ang [1-9] by ACE2. Thus, under physiological conditions, ACE2 mainly forms Ang [1-7] than Ang [1-9] [34].

While Ang II, which acts via angiotensin 1/AT1 [primary mediator] and angiotensin 2/AT2 receptors is a potent vasoconstrictor, a pro-fibrotic, and a pro-inflammatory agent, Ang [1-7] acts via Mas receptors and has vasodilator, anti-apoptotic and anti-proliferative effect. Mas receptors are G protein-coupled receptors and in the brain, they are highly expressed in the dentate gyrus of the hippocampus, a site-specific for adult neurogenesis and in blood vessels [35]. The ACE2/Ang [1-7]/Mas receptor axis of the RAS is considered to be the protective arm of the renin-angiotensin system. A balance in ACE/ACE2 is critical which implies a balance between the pro-inflammatory pro-oxidative arm and the anti-inflammatory and anti-oxidative arm of RAS. An increase in ACE/ACE2 ratio was observed in many pathological conditions including cardiovascular pathology, renal dysfunction, pulmonary hypertension, in cigarette smokers, and Alzheimer's disease [36–39]. SARS-CoV-2 which enters the host cells via ACE2 also causes downregulation of ACE2 and the major targets of SARS-CoV-2 are those which express higher levels of ACE2 [26]. The fibrotic and inflammatory processes observed in various organs in COVID-19 patients could be attributed to the dysregulation of ACE2 and subsequently, RAS which is observed in endocrine, paracrine, and intracrine levels in several organs [40]. Dysregulation of RAS in the brain is associated with neuroinflammation and neurodegeneration [41].

5. Neurogenesis

The old dogma that the production of functional neurons does not occur in adult life was refuted when Altman and Das published evidence to support the

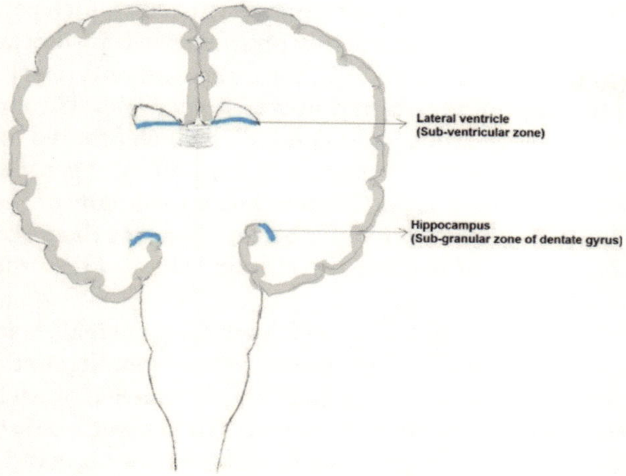

Figure 3.
Coronal section of the brain showing the sites of adult neurogenesis.

continuation of neurogenesis in adult life in rodents [42]. Neurogenesis refers to the process of the generation of new neurons from neural stem cells. This process which plays a major role in brain development in embryonic life ceases to exist shortly after birth in the majority of brain areas except two. The subgranular zone [SGZ] of the dentate gyrus of the hippocampus and subventricular zone [SVZ], lining the lateral wall of the lateral ventricles are the two areas where neurogenesis persists well into adult life albeit declining slightly with ageing (**Figure 3**) [43, 44]. There is a complex microenvironment that nourishes and supports the neural progenitor cells and their progeny which is called the 'neurogenic niche'. There are various trophic factors, blood vessels, supporting glial cells, and hormones in the neurogenic niche that help to control and enhance neurogenesis [45]. The newborn neurons mature and get integrated into neural circuits and are involved in a variety of functions including learning and memory like temporal and pattern separation, high-resolution memory, synaptic plasticity, fear conditioning and emotions, and olfaction [46]. Incidentally altered neurogenesis is implicated in several neuropsychiatric diseases like Alzheimer's disease, Parkinson's disease, depression, Huntington's disease, and stroke, epilepsy, and demyelinating disease [46, 47].

5.1 Stages of adult neurogenesis

The process of adult neurogenesis occurs in stages viz. maintenance of neural stem/progenitor cells [NPC] and proliferation of NPC, fate specification/commitment, differentiation, maturation, survival of immature neurons, and integration into neural circuitry. The defining abilities of NPC are self-replication and multipotency, that is, the ability to differentiate into multiple lineages of cells and in this case neurons, astrocytes, and oligodendrocytes [48]. There are different types of neural progenitor cells in SGZ and SVZ. Type-1 cells in SGZ, B-cells in SVZ, and radial glia-like cells in SGZ and SVZ are largely quiescent cells, which are similar to radial glia cells found during embryonic development and have a morphology similar to mature astrocytes. Type-2 cells in SGZ and C-cells in SVZ are small roundish cells that are highly proliferative, and they give rise to type-3 cells in SGZ and A-cells in SVZ which represent committed neuroblasts. The type-1/B-cells are multipotent and have unlimited self-renewal capacity which get activated by various factors and multiply to form highly proliferative transient intermediate progenitor cells [TIP] in the SGZ. In SVZ, the transit-amplifying cells [TAC] [type-2/C-cells] has the ability to differentiate into neurons. These divide to form neuroblasts or immature neurons [type-3/A-cells] which proceed to neuronal differentiation and forms newborn neurons that mature and get integrated into neural circuitry in the brain. It is pertinent to know that many of the newborn neurons perish and only 15–30% of immature neurons survive the maturation process. There are various factors that regulate this step and thereby the process of adult neurogenesis [49–51].

In SGZ, the NPCs form granule cells which are the principal excitatory cells of the dentate gyrus. Their axons form the mossy fibres extending to the CA3 region and their dendrites are in the molecular layer which receives connections from the entorhinal cortex. Immature neurons that are less than a week-old start to have neurite outgrowth and by one- or two-weeks axons can be observed in the hilus, and dendrites start to extend to the molecular layer without spines which being developed by around the 16th day. By 17 days, functional connections are formed by the axons [mossy fibres] with the CA3 pyramidal neurons [52]. They release glutamate as the neurotransmitter. After around 1 week of birth, the newborn granule cells receive GABAergic inputs and after 2 weeks receive glutamatergic inputs [53]. These immature neurons exhibit enhanced excitability by virtue of high input resistance and subthreshold calcium ion conductance which enables them to develop action potential with less excitatory currents. They also have a low threshold for induction of LTP [long-term potentiation] [54, 55]. Between 3 weeks and 2 months, there occurs a gradual increase in spine formation, dendritic arborisation and connection, boutons on CA3 neurons, and maturation of mossy fibres. By less than 2 months, the newborn neurons become functionally indistinguishable from fully mature granule cells [52].

Intrinsic factors	Examples
Neurotrophic factors	brain-derived neurotrophic factor (BDNF), insulin-like growth factor-1 (IGF-1), nerve growth factor (NGF), glia-derived nerve factor (GDNF), fibroblast growth factor 2 (FGF-2), epidermal growth factor (EGF)
Morphogens	Notch, sonic hedgehog (Shh), wingless ligands (Wnts), and bone morphogenic proteins (BMPs).
Inflammatory cytokines	tissue necrosis factors α (TNFα), interleukin-6 (IL-6) and IL-1β IL-4 and IL-10
Neurotransmitters	gamma-aminobutyric acid (GABA), glutamate, dopamine, serotonin, norepinephrine, acetylcholine
Hormones	Glucocorticoids, sex hormones, leptin, incretin
Epigenetic factors	methyl-CpG-binding domain protein 1 (Mbd1), MYST family histone acetyltransferase Querkopf (Qkf), mixed-lineage leukaemia 1 (Mll1), polycomb complex protein (Bmi-1), histone deacetylase 2 (HDAC2), and microRNAs (miR124, 137, 184, 185, and 491-3p)
Transcriptional factors	sex-determining region Y-box 2 (Sox2), Orphan nuclear receptor TLX, forkhead box O proteins (FoxOs), prospero homeobox 1 (Prox1), neurogenic differentiation1 (NeuroD1), Kruppel-like factor 9, cyclic AMP response element-binding protein (CREB), paired box protein (Pax6), and neurogenin 2 (Neurog2)

Table 3.
List of intrinsic factors that affect adult neurogenesis.

In SVZ, restricted neural progenitor cells migrate along scaffolds maintained by specialised astrocytes via the rostral migratory stream [RMS] to reach the olfactory bulb. By 15–30 days, they differentiate into two types of interneurons, GABAergic granule neurons [95%] and GABA or dopaminergic periglomerular neurons [5%]. The newborn GABAergic granule neurons can become cells with dendrites that do not cross beyond the mitral cell layer and those with non-spiny dendrites that extend till the external plexiform layer. These interneurons mature and get integrated into olfactory network and start responding to olfactory signals [52].

There are various factors that regulate neurogenesis. These include intrinsic niche-derived intrinsic mechanisms and extrinsic systemic factors. The intrinsic factors that regulate adult neurogenesis are given in **Table 3**. There are extrinsic environmental cues and systemic factors that can positively and negatively affect adult neurogenesis like physical exercise, dietary intake, olfactory/hippocampal-dependent learning, environmental enrichment, ageing, stress, alcohol abuse, and certain inflammatory conditions [46, 56–59].

6. Entry of SARS-CoV-2 into the brain

There are different ways that are the possible pathway for the entry of SARS-CoV-2 into the brain. Some of the ways include olfactory transmucosal invasion, hematogenous dissemination, and neuronal retrograde dissemination [5]. The olfactory sensory neurons of the olfactory mucosa are bipolar neurons. The axons of the olfactory sensory neurons along the apical side project into the nasal cavity while that on the basal side merge into filia and protrudes into the olfactory bulb through the cribriform plate. Thus, the olfactory sensory neurons are in direct contact with the cerebrospinal fluid [60]. In the olfactory mucosa, ACE2 receptors are mainly found in the non-neuronal cells, sustentacular cells while their expression in the olfactory sensory neurons is less [30]. The blood vessels lining the olfactory mucosa express both ACE2 and TMPRSS2 protease receptors which help in the invasion of the SARS-CoV-2 virus and facilitate binding, replication, and accumulation of the virus [61, 62]. Studies have found that SARS-CoV-2 enters CNS through this neural-mucosal interface by infection of the olfactory neurons or by diffusion through channels formed by olfactory ensheathing cells in the olfactory mucosa [60, 63]. Following the olfactory transmucosal invasion, the virus passes along the olfactory tract via axonal transport, trans-synaptic transport, or microfusion to different areas of the brain linked with the olfactory tract [60, 64].

Recent studies have observed that SARS-CoV-2 RNA was found in brain regions that are not directly connected to olfactory mucosa like the cerebellum which shows that other forms/routes of viral entry into the brain are at play. Neuronal retrograde dissemination is the one where the virus may breach peripheral nerve terminals and take a trans-synaptic route to reach CNS. For instance, SARS-CoV-2 may invade peripheral chemoreceptors and may reach the cardiorespiratory centre in the brain stem [65] or through the gut-brain axis where the virus may enter the brain through enteric nerves [66]. In case of hematogenous dissemination, the virus after infecting the airways may breach the epithelial barrier and enter the bloodstream. Through systemic circulation, the virus may reach the cerebral circulation and could infect endothelial cells of blood–brain barrier or epithelial cells of the blood CSF barrier to reach the brain or via circumventricular organs which lack the blood–brain barrier [5]. Trojan horse mechanism is another way by which SARS-CoV-2 could reach the brain parenchyma. It is the process in which the virus infects leucocytes which get activated and disseminate to other tissues and cross blood–brain barrier [67].

Once SARS-CoV-2 enters the brain, it enters and infects the neurons, glial cells, and endothelial cells through ACE2 and replicates which leads to cell death. It causes damage to the blood–brain barrier which will increase its permeability and cause oedema, intracerebral bleeding, and neuronal death. The infected neurons can release inflammatory mediators that can activate other immune cells like mast cells, neurons, microglia, astrocytes, endothelial cells, and pericytes [68, 69].

7. Adult neurogenesis in COVID-19

Earlier studies show that survivors of critical illness have higher risk of developing neuropsychiatric consequences after discharge from the hospital. The prevalence of symptoms of depression, anxiety, and post-traumatic stress was found to be 29% [28–34], 34% [30–42], and 34% [27–50] in survivors of critical illness, respectively [70–72]. Impairment in memory, attention, and concentration was observed in SARS survivors 1 year after recovery [73]. Based on the knowledge from earlier infections by coronaviruses, SARS, and MERS, an increased risk of neuropsychiatric disorders like depression, anxiety, post-traumatic stress disorder, are possible in a long-term follow-up of patients recovered from COVID-19 [12].

Neuropsychiatric disorders that display impaired adult neurogenesis include major depressive disorder, Alzheimer's disease, Parkinson's disease, schizophrenia, and post-traumatic stress disorder. All of these correlate well with the reduction in hippocampal volume, cognitive deficits, and mood dysregulation [74]. A recent 3-month prospective study by Yiping Lu et al. conducted in COVID-19 recovered patients found that there was grey matter enlargement in olfactory cortices and hippocampus bilaterally [75]. Yiping Lu et al. also found that the grey matter volume of the hippocampus was negatively related to loss of smell during the disease phase [75]. Anosmia over a course of time in upper respiratory tract infections was found to be associated with a decrease in the grey matter volume [GMV] of the central olfactory system due to loss of stimulation while enlargement of GMV is observed during recovery [76]. Functional compensation in the form of enlarged neurons and an increase in the dendritic spine and compensatory enhanced neurogenesis are believed to be the reason behind GMV enlargement during recovery [77]. Loss of memory that persisted 3 months after the active infection in COVID-19 recovered patients was found to be negatively related to hippocampal grey matter volume [75]. Memory acquisition depends on newborn neurons and impairment in the acquisition of memory occurs due to inhibition of adult neurogenesis in the hippocampus [78, 79].

Anosmia is regarded as the key feature of COVID-19 which either occurs as an only symptom or in association with other signs and symptoms [80, 81]. Earlier studies show that any impairment in olfactory neurogenesis is associated with anosmia since neurogenesis in the olfactory epithelium and olfactory bulb is essential for the sense of smell [82, 83]. Dysfunction or atrophy of the olfactory bulb was observed in COVID-19 patients by recent studies done using brain imaging reports [84, 85]. Pathogenic changes in COVID-19 seem to cause loss of dopaminergic neurons, defects in the dopamine system, and exacerbate the clinical features of Parkinson's disease [PD] [86, 87]. Anosmia is an important premotor symptom of PD which is not directly related to the neurodegenerative process in substantia nigra but appears to be related to defective adult neurogenesis [88, 89].

Understanding the process of adult neurogenesis in COVID-19 may reveal a critical role of the regenerative capacity of NPCs in combating the neuropsychiatric consequence of COVID-19. There are no studies or evidence to link COVID-19 with adult neurogenesis yet. Based on the factors like the presentation of neuropsychiatric symptoms in COVID-19, the occurrence of symptoms like anosmia, memory and cognitive deficits in COVID-19, the neuro-invasive potential of SARS-CoV-2, ACE2 expression in sites of adult neurogenesis, increased levels of pro-inflammatory cytokines like IL-6, Il-1β which inhibit adult neurogenesis and impact of earlier coronavirus infections, it might not be far-fetched to say that COVID-19 could have a possible impact on adult neurogenesis. There is a severe scarcity in research analysing the effect of SARS-CoV-2 infection on adult neurogenesis. The current chapter, which is speculative and based on a thorough literature search, discusses the possible changes in adult neurogenesis in COVID-19 emphasising the role of ACE2. If proven to be true in the future, the findings in this article will help in achieving early intervention to address the neuropsychiatric long-term consequence of COVID-19.

8. Role of ACE2 in adult neurogenesis in COVID-19

SARS-CoV-2 entry into the cell through ACE2 is followed by the downregulation of ACE2. A decrease in ACE2 will lead to dysregulation of RAS and various other complications. A recent study has found that ACE2 is expressed in young neurons and in human-induced pluripotent stem cell-derived neural progenitor cells [90]. ACE2 is found to have various neuroprotective functions. It converts neurotoxic amyloid protein Aβ into neuroprotective one in transgenic mice [91]. ACE2 activator, diminazene increased CREB, BDNF, glutamate, and nicotinic receptor and decreased the levels of apoptotic and inflammatory proteins in the AD model of D-galactose-ovariectomized rats [92]. All these factors play a major role in adult neurogenesis. ACE2 deficiency in mice was found to be accompanied by significantly impaired learning and memory [93]. Exercise-induced neurogenesis in the dentate gyrus was abolished in ACE2 deficient mice. Ang II, Ang [1-7], and Mas receptors were not found to be responsible and hence the mediator of this effect is not identified yet [94].

ACE2 expression is stronger in the enterocytes of the small intestine and colon, which is even higher than in the lungs. Neural ganglia cells in the colon of the enteric nervous system also express ACE2 receptors. Intestinal ACE2 plays a major role in the transport of neutral amino acids via B0AT1, neutral amino acid transporter. ACE2/B0AT1 complex regulates the composition and function of gut microbiota. ACE2 knockout animals showed lower levels of serum neutral amino acid levels like tryptophan, and impaired gut microbiota composition along with reduced expression of small intestinal antimicrobial peptides [95]. Enteric infection is an important presentation of COVID-19. Faeces of COVID-19 patients were found to have Viral mRNA [96, 97]. SARS-CoV-2 entry via the enteric route into host cell leads to ACE2 shedding due to S priming which may lead to gut microbiota dysbiosis [98]. Depletion of gut microbiota by prolonged antibiotic treatment resulted in impairment in cognitive function and hippocampal neurogenesis in adult mice [99]. The existence of a strong link between gut microbiota and the development of mental disorders, depression, and anxiety which are associated with impaired adult neurogenesis has been explored in recent studies [100].

Neuroinflammation directly impairs adult hippocampal neurogenesis. Pro-inflammatory cytokine IL-1β, IL-6, IFN-α causes a reduction in neural cell proliferation and suppresses adult hippocampal neurogenesis [101–103]. SARS-CoV-2 entry into the brain triggers an immune response by activating microglia, astrocytes, and other immune cells. This leads to increased production of cytokines in the brain. Cytokine storm which is a deadly hyperinflammatory response is considered to be a hallmark feature of COVID-19 pathogenesis [104]. Hypercytokinemia of IL-6, IL-10, and TNF-α was observed in COVID-19 patients. Increased levels of IL-6 correlate with mortality and the need for ventilator support [105, 106].

Thus, there are different possible mechanisms through which SARS-CoV-2 affects adult neurogenesis via ACE2. This chapter, however, will focus on the role of ACE2 in possible alterations in adult neurogenesis in COVID-19 via neurotransmitters.

9. ACE2 and neurotransmitters involved in adult neurogenesis

Neurotransmitter signalling is found to play a major role in the formation of new neurons in addition to its clear and indisputable role in communication between neurons. Starting from embryogenesis, neurotransmitters are involved in neuronal proliferation. In adult neurogenesis, they influence various steps including proliferation, differentiation, and migration. In addition to the direct action of neurotransmitters on adult neurogenesis, they also influence other factors that regulate neurogenesis like neurotrophic factors and growth factors [107].

9.1 ACE2 and serotonin

Serotonin is a crucial monoaminergic neurotransmitter that acts as a mood stabiliser and is associated with feelings of happiness, well-being, and contentedness. In the brain, it is synthesised by the Raphe nuclei neurons in the brain stem from tryptophan using neuron-specific tryptophan hydroxylase 2 enzymes. Vesicular monoamine transporter 2 [VMAT] packs the synthesised serotonin into vesicles. Serotonin transporters [SERT] re-uptake serotonin back to presynaptic neurons after its release, thereby regulating its extracellular levels [108]. The serotonergic fibres from raphe nuclei have projections throughout the brain and especially to the granule cells and interneurons of the dentate gyrus of the hippocampus. Serotonin is known to play a major regulatory role in adult hippocampal neurogenesis. Selective serotonin reuptake inhibitors [SRRI] are commonly used antidepressants that act by increasing serotonin levels in the brain causes clinical improvement associated with an increase in adult hippocampal neurogenesis characterised by increased neuronal proliferation and number of newborn neurons [109]. Malberg et al. in 2000 were the first to show that chronic treatment with fluoxetine improved adult hippocampal neurogenesis [109]. In the dentate gyrus, serotonin is known to promote neuronal development and its depletion was found to cause reduced dendritic spine density of granule cells [110–113]. Chronic treatment with SSRI, fluoxetine was found to increase the survival of newborn neurons in the dentate gyrus [109, 114]. In stress models like inescapable stress, cold restraint stress in the animal model, fluoxetine administration was found to exhibit neurogenic and neuroprotective roles in the hippocampus [114, 115]. Accelerated synaptogenesis and increased long-term potentiation [LTP] in the hippocampus were also observed by long-term treatment by fluoxetine [116].

Recent studies have found that ACE2 plays a major role in the biosynthesis of serotonin [5HT]. The precursor for 5HT is an essential amino acid, tryptophan which can cross the blood–brain barrier and whose intestinal absorption was found to be reduced by 70% in case of ACE2 deficiency. Thus, ACE2 has an indirect modulatory role in 5HT synthesis in the brain [117]. There are recent studies that show that 5HT synthesis in the brain is dependent on ACE2, which acts by modulating 5HT metabolism and ACE2 deficiency leads to decreased serum tryptophan levels and decreased serotonin levels in the brain [94].

9.2 ACE2 and dopamine

Dopamine is involved in executive functions, volition, motor control, motivation, pleasure/reward, and attention/concentration [118]. The role and mechanism of action of dopamine in adult neurogenesis are not elucidated fully. Dopamine was found to modulate cell proliferation in the embryonic brain [119]. Hippocampus and sub-ventricular zone [SVZ] which are the neurogenic niche containing neural stem cells receive dopaminergic projections from the substantia nigra and ventral tegmental area. Dopamine receptors are also widely expressed in these two areas and play a regulatory role in adult neurogenesis and neural plasticity [120, 121]. Earlier studies show that depletion of dopamine in the rat model reduces both proliferation and survival of neural precursor cells in the sub-granular zone [SGZ] of the dentate gyrus [122, 123]. Dopaminergic denervation in substantia nigra caused a significant reduction in the proliferation of neural stem cells in SGZ and SVZ which was reversed by D2 receptor stimulation in rodents [123]. In humans, post-mortem studies have revealed that the number of neural precursor cells in SGZ and SVZ was reduced in patients with Parkinson's disease [124]. Dopamine was also found to increase the type 2A early progenitor cell in the hippocampus of rodents via D1 like receptors [118]. Dopamine receptor agonist pramipexole increases the proliferation and survival of newborn neurons in SVZ, olfactory bulb [119].

RAS plays a major role in dopaminergic vulnerability through AT1 receptors. Dysregulation of RAS due to the downregulation of ACE2 induced by SARS-CoV-2 may increase the vulnerability of dopaminergic neurons and subsequently dopamine levels [125]. Interactions between dopamine and angiotensin receptors that are counterregulatory in nature are observed in substantia nigra and striatum [125]. The gene for ACE2 was found to coexpress and coregulate with that of dopa decarboxylase [DDC] in non-neuronal cells, which is a major enzyme of dopamine, serotonin, and histamine biosynthesis. DDC converts L-3,4-dihydroxyphenylalanine [L-DOPA] into dopamine which subsequently forms norepinephrine and epinephrine and L-5-hydroxytryptophan into serotonin. This coexpression and coregulation link between the genes for ACE2 and DDC gives rise to the possibility of a functional link between the actions of ACE2 and DDC [i.e.,] in the synthesis of Ang [1-7] and dopamine and serotonin mediated by ACE2 and DDC, respectively [126]. Following the infusion of Ang [1-7] in the hypothalamus of rats, brain dopamine levels increased which emphasises the link between ACE2 and DDC. SARS-CoV-2 induced downregulation of ACE2 could cause the decreased synthesis of serotonin and dopamine [94, 127].

The SARS-CoV-2 infection has been found to cause loss of dopaminergic neurons and deficits in the dopamine system [86, 128]. ACE2 expression is high in dopaminergic neurons and the downregulation of ACE2 by SARS-CoV-2 may cause depletion of dopaminergic neurons and dopamine levels. This is evident from the worsening of symptoms observed in COVID-19 patients with Parkinson's disease [PD], requiring increased dopamine replacement therapy [129]. ACE2 deletion in the knockout mouse model caused a significant reduction in dopamine D1 mRNA expression in substantia nigra [130].

9.3 ACE2 and norepinephrine

Norepinephrine is an important catecholamine that is involved in alertness, arousal, sleep–wake cycle, memory storage, and emotions. It modulates various functions of the hippocampus like learning, memory, and mood. Noradrenergic axon terminals arising from the locus coeruleus densely innervate the neurogenic niche in the adult hippocampus [131]. Norepinephrine along with the other monoaminergic neurotransmitters plays a major role in adult neurogenesis. Norepinephrine was found to activate the stem cells and neural precursor cells via β3-adrenergic receptors where non-proliferating latent precursor cells develop the ability to respond to mitogens and generate neurospheres. It also increases the proliferation of early progenitor cells in the adult hippocampus via β2-adrenergic receptors [132, 133]. Depletion of norepinephrine significantly decreased the proliferation of progenitor cells of granule cells in the hippocampus [134]. Antidepressants that selectively increase norepinephrine were found to increase adult hippocampal neurogenesis [132].

Downregulation of ACE2 by SARS-CoV-2 may affect the activity of DDC due to the coexpression and coregulation between the genes for ACE2 and DDC. This could lead to a decrease in the biosynthesis of dopamine and subsequently norepinephrine [126].

9.4 ACE2 and glutamate and GABA

Glutamate is the predominant excitatory neurotransmitter of the CNS. It plays a vital role in both embryonic brain development and adult neurogenesis. Its extracellular levels are especially higher in the neurogenic niche when compared to other areas of the brain [135, 136]. It has trophic effects on the developing neurons before synapse formation like proliferation, migration, and maturation. It causes an increase in the proliferation of neural progenitor cells [NPC]. The NPCs express NMDA metabotropic glutamate receptors, stimulation of which caused increased intracellular calcium and activation of NeuroD1, proneural gene [137]. Glutamate signalling plays a positive role in maintaining the proliferation of NPCs and the survival rates of newborn neurons [137, 138].

Gamma-aminobutyric acid [GABA] is a principal inhibitory neurotransmitter in the CNS. It is produced from glutamate by the action of the enzymes glutamate decarboxylase GAD65 and GAD67 [139]. Dysfunction in the GABAergic system is implicated in major depressive disorder and anxiety [140]. However, in the developing brain, GABA exerts an excitatory effect, that is, GABA is excitatory in immature neurons. Tonic discharge from GABAergic neurons is necessary for maintaining the quiescent state of NPCs. The absence of GABAergic excitability will cause impairment in neuronal maturation and synapse formation while an excess of it over newborn neurons will lead to seizures [141]. In SGZ, GABA mediates depolarisation of progenitor cells which is involved in the incorporation of AMPA receptors in immature granule cells, which is critical for learning and formation of memory [142]. It has a negative influence on neuroblasts. It inhibits the proliferation and migration of neuroblasts. It also inhibits the proliferation of NPCs [143–145]. It also promotes the differentiation of hippocampal NPCs. GABAA receptor agonist, phenobarbital caused a reduction in NPC proliferation and increase in differentiation which resulted in an increased number of newborn neurons [146]. Thus, it plays crucial role in different stages of adult neurogenesis. GABA and glutamate signalling play a major role in adult neurogenesis. Selective activation of the receptor subtypes of GABA and glutamate expressed in NPCs plays a pivotal role in self-replication and fate commitment of the developing neurons into a particular progeny [147].

A recent study has found ACE2 to be located mainly in excitatory neurons of the brain and to a lesser extent in inhibitory neurons like GABAergic neurons [148]. This indicates that SARS-CoV-2 once enters the brain has the potential to access the glutamatergic and GABAergic neurons. The consequence of this is not known however, viral entry may trigger apoptotic pathways and cause excitatory-inhibitory imbalance, and lead to neuronal death [149]. Cytokine release from infected neurons and other activated microglia and astrocytes may also cause a decrease in glutamate and GABA [150]. These effects are implicated along with impaired adult neurogenesis in neurodegenerative diseases like Parkinson's disease and Alzheimer's disease. Seizure is one of the neurological symptoms in COVID-19 patients, in which an increase in glutamate levels and decrease in GABA levels in the cerebral cortex and hippocampus is an implicated mechanism [151]. This further emphasises the possible impact of SARS-CoV-2 on glutamate and GABA.

Thus, SARS-CoV-2 induced downregulation of ACE2 in COVID-19 is potentially detrimental to adult neurogenesis. ACE2 deficiency affects the levels and actions of the neurotransmitters serotonin, dopamine, norepinephrine, GABA, and glutamate which play crucial roles in adult neurogenesis.

10. Conclusion

SARS-CoV-2 has been found to have a high affinity to ACE2 receptors. Such high affinity has been linked to affect neurogenesis through a variety of mechanisms. The present chapter has clearly postulated the link between this deadly virus and its effect on monoaminergic neurotransmitters as well as GABA and glutamate which play a major role in adult neurogenesis. As ACE2 receptors are expressed in the hippocampus, decreased neurogenesis in this region could be one of the major factors behind the neuropsychiatric disorders associated with patients affected with COVID-19. Awareness and early intervention to prevent and treat long-term psychiatric consequences of COVID-19 are crucial. We should be aware of the possibility that in the long term, COVID-19 may be associated with cognitive and psychiatric disorders in those who recovered. Despite having a mild course of disease in children and adolescents, immunological response to the infection in this population may affect synaptic pruning which may lead to various issues that may not be immediately apparent. Insights into the various machinations of adult neurogenesis in COVID-19 can be used to engineer the process to help with the pathological changes in the brain inflicted by the disease.

Acknowledgements

The authors would like to thank the Deanship of Scientific Research, Majmaah University for the support of this chapter.

Author details

Jayakumar Saikarthik[1], Ilango Saraswathi[2*] and Abdulrahman A. Al-Atram[3]

1 Department of Basic Medical Sciences, Department of Medical Education, College of Dentistry, Majmaah University, Al Majmaah, Riyadh, Saudi Arabia

2 Madha Medical College and Research Institute, Chennai, India

3 College of Medicine, Majmaah University, Al Majmaah, Riyadh, Saudi Arabia

*Address all correspondence to: saraswathiddentistt@gmail.com

References

[1] Worldometer. Worldometer Coronavirus. United States: Dadax Limited; 2021. Available from: https://www.worldometers.info/coronavirus/

[2] WHO. Archived: WHO Timeline—COVID-19. Geneva: WHO; 2020 Available from: https://www.who.int/news/item/27-04-2020-who-timeline---covid-19

[3] Wang S, Ye J, Kang Z, Peng H, Mackey V, Sun L. The COVID-19 pandemic and the potential treatment of the novel coronavirus SARS-CoV-2. American Journal of Translational Research. 2021;**13**(3):871

[4] CDC. COVID-19; Symptoms of COVID-19. United Kingdom: CDC; 2020 Available from: https://www.cdc.gov/coronavirus/2019-ncov/symptoms-testing/symptoms.html [Accessed: 22 February 2021]

[5] Pezzini A, Padovani A. Lifting the mask on neurological manifestations of COVID-19. Nature Reviews Neurology. 2020;**16**(11):636-644

[6] Desai I, Manchanda R, Kumar N, Tiwari A, Kumar M. Neurological manifestations of coronavirus disease 2019: Exploring past to understand present. Neurological Sciences. 2021;**42**(3):773-785

[7] Huang C, Wang Y, Li X, Ren L, Zhao J, Hu Y, et al. Clinical features of patients infected with 2019 novel coronavirus in Wuhan, China. The Lancet. 2020;**395**(10223):497-506

[8] Cardona GC, Pájaro LDQ, Marzola IDQ, Villegas YR, Salazar LRM. Neurotropism of SARS-CoV 2: Mechanisms and manifestations. Journal of the Neurological Sciences. 2020;**412**:116824

[9] Moriguchi T, Harii N, Goto J, Harada D, Sugawara H, Takamino J, et al. A first case of meningitis/encephalitis associated with SARS-Coronavirus-2. International Journal of Infectious Diseases. 2020;**94**:55-58

[10] Chu H, Chan JF-W, Yuen TT-T, Shuai H, Yuan S, Wang Y, et al. Comparative tropism, replication kinetics, and cell damage profiling of SARS-CoV-2 and SARS-CoV with implications for clinical manifestations, transmissibility, and laboratory studies of COVID-19: An observational study. The Lancet Microbe. 2020;**1**(1):e14-e23

[11] Arbour N, Day R, Newcombe J, Talbot PJ. Neuroinvasion by human respiratory coronaviruses. Journal of Virology. 2000;**74**(19):8913-8921

[12] Rogers JP, Chesney E, Oliver D, Pollak TA, McGuire P, Fusar-Poli P, et al. Psychiatric and neuropsychiatric presentations associated with severe coronavirus infections: A systematic review and meta-analysis with comparison to the COVID-19 pandemic. The Lancet Psychiatry. 2020;**7**(7):611-627

[13] Corman V, Lienau J, Witzenrath M. Coronaviruses as the cause of respiratory infections. Der Internist. 2019;**60**(11):1136-1145

[14] Hewings-Martin Y. How do SARS and MERS compare with COVID-19? United Kingdom: MedicalNewsToday; 2020

[15] Gallagher TM, Buchmeier MJ. Coronavirus spike proteins in viral entry and pathogenesis. Virology. 2001;**279**(2):371-374

[16] Hoffmann M, Kleine-Weber H, Schroeder S, Krüger N, Herrler T, Erichsen S, et al. SARS-CoV-2 cell entry depends on ACE2 and TMPRSS2 and is blocked by a clinically proven protease inhibitor. Cell. 2020;**181**(2):271-80.e8

[17] Coutard B, Valle C, de Lamballerie X, Canard B, Seidah NG, Decroly E. The spike glycoprotein of the new coronavirus 2019-nCoV contains a furin-like cleavage site absent in CoV of the same clade. Antiviral Research. 2020;**176**:104742

[18] Wrapp D, Wang N, Corbett KS, Goldsmith JA, Hsieh C-L, Abiona O, et al. Cryo-EM structure of the 2019-nCoV spike in the prefusion conformation. Science. 2020;**367**(6483): 1260-1263

[19] Donoghue M, Hsieh F, Baronas E, Godbout K, Gosselin M, Stagliano N, et al. A novel angiotensin-converting enzyme–related carboxypeptidase [ACE2] converts angiotensin I to angiotensin 1-9. Circulation Research. 2000;**87**(5):e1-e9

[20] Tipnis SR, Hooper NM, Hyde R, Karran E, Christie G, Turner AJ. A human homolog of angiotensin-converting enzyme: Cloning and functional expression as a captopril-insensitive carboxypeptidase. Journal of Biological Chemistry. 2000;**275**(43): 33238-33243

[21] Gheblawi M, Wang K, Viveiros A, Nguyen Q, Zhong J-C, Turner AJ, et al. Angiotensin-converting enzyme 2: SARS-CoV-2 receptor and regulator of the renin-angiotensin system: Celebrating the 20th anniversary of the discovery of ACE2. Circulation Research. 2020;**126**(10):1456-1474

[22] Kalea AZ, Batlle D. Apelin and ACE2 in cardiovascular disease. Current Opinion in Investigational Drugs. 2010;**11**(3):273-282

[23] Vickers C, Hales P, Kaushik V, Dick L, Gavin J, Tang J, et al. Hydrolysis of biological peptides by human angiotensin-converting enzyme-related carboxypeptidase. Journal of Biological Chemistry. 2002;**277**(17):14838-14843

[24] Warner FJ, Lew RA, Smith AI, Lambert DW, Hooper NM, Turner AJ. Angiotensin-converting enzyme 2 [ACE2], but not ACE, is preferentially localized to the apical surface of polarized kidney cells. Journal of Biological Chemistry. 2005;**280**(47): 39353-39362

[25] Clarke NE, Turner AJ. Angiotensin-converting enzyme 2: The first decade. International Journal of Hypertension. 2012;**2012**:307315

[26] Pagliaro P, Penna C. ACE/ACE2 ratio: A key also in 2019 coronavirus disease [Covid-19]? Frontiers in Medicine. 2020;**7**(335):1-5

[27] Danilczyk U, Eriksson U, Crackower MA, Penninger JM. A story of two ACEs. Journal of Molecular Medicine. 2003;**81**(4):227-234

[28] Walls AC, Park Y-J, Tortorici MA, Wall A, McGuire AT, Veesler D. Structure, function, and antigenicity of the SARS-CoV-2 spike glycoprotein. Cell. 2020;**181**(2):281-92.e6

[29] Hernández VS, Zetter MA, Guerra EC, Hernández-Araiza I, Karuzin N, Hernández-Pérez OR, et al. ACE2 expression in rat brain: Implications for COVID-19 associated neurological manifestations. bioRxiv. 2021:2021.05.01.442293

[30] Bilinska K, Jakubowska P, Von Bartheld CS, Butowt R. Expression of the SARS-CoV-2 entry proteins, ACE2 and TMPRSS2, in cells of the olfactory epithelium: Identification of cell types and trends with age. ACS Chemical Neuroscience. 2020;**11**(11):1555-1562

[31] Hamming I, Timens W, Bulthuis M, Lely A, Gv N, van Goor H. Tissue distribution of ACE2 protein, the functional receptor for SARS coronavirus. A first step in understanding SARS pathogenesis. The Journal of Pathology: A Journal of the Pathological Society of Great Britain and Ireland. 2004;**203**(2):631-637

[32] Alenina N, Bader M. ACE2 in brain physiology and pathophysiology: Evidence from transgenic animal models. Neurochemical Research. 2019;**44**(6):1323-1329

[33] Silva RAP, Chu Y, Miller JD, Mitchell IJ, Penninger JM, Faraci FM, et al. Impact of ACE2 deficiency and oxidative stress on cerebrovascular function with aging. Stroke. 2012; **43**(12):3358-3363

[34] Rice GI, Thomas DA, Grant PJ, Turner AJ, Hooper NM. Evaluation of angiotensin-converting enzyme [ACE], its homologue ACE2 and neprilysin in angiotensin peptide metabolism. Biochemical Journal. 2004;**383**(1):45-51

[35] Hellner K, Walther T, Schubert M, Albrecht D. Angiotensin-[1-7] enhances LTP in the hippocampus through the G-protein-coupled receptor Mas. Molecular and Cellular Neuroscience. 2005;**29**(3):427-435

[36] Bernardi S, Toffoli B, Zennaro C, Tikellis C, Monticone S, Losurdo P, et al. High-salt diet increases glomerular ACE/ACE2 ratio leading to oxidative stress and kidney damage. Nephrology Dialysis Transplantation. 2012;**27**(5): 1793-1800

[37] Lavrentyev EN, Malik KU. High glucose-induced Nox1-derived superoxides downregulate PKC-βII, which subsequently decreases ACE2 expression and ANG [1-7] formation in rat VSMCs. American Journal of Physiology-Heart and Circulatory Physiology. 2009;**296**(1):H106-HH18

[38] Yuan Y-M, Luo L, Guo Z, Yang M, Ye R-S, Luo C. Activation of renin–angiotensin–aldosterone system [RAAS] in the lung of smoking-induced pulmonary arterial hypertension [PAH] rats. Journal of the Renin-Angiotensin-Aldosterone System. 2015;**16**(2):249-253

[39] Kehoe PG, Wong S, Mulhim NA, Palmer LE, Miners JS. Angiotensin-converting enzyme 2 is reduced in Alzheimer's disease in association with increasing amyloid-β and tau pathology. Alzheimer's Research & Therapy. 2016;**8**(1):1-10

[40] Valenzuela R, Rodriguez-Perez AI, Costa-Besada MA, Rivas-Santisteban R, Garrido-Gil P, Lopez-Lopez A, et al. An ACE2/Mas-related receptor MrgE axis in dopaminergic neuron mitochondria. Redox Biology. 2021;**46**:102078

[41] Labandeira-García JL, Garrido-Gil P, Rodriguez-Pallares J, Valenzuela R, Borrajo A, Rodríguez-Perez AI. Brain renin-angiotensin system and dopaminergic cell vulnerability. Frontiers in Neuroanatomy. 2014;**8**:67

[42] Altman J, Das GD. Autoradiographic and histological evidence of postnatal hippocampal neurogenesis in rats. Journal of Comparative Neurology. 1965;**124**(3):319-335

[43] Taverna E, Götz M, Huttner WB. The cell biology of neurogenesis: Toward an understanding of the development and evolution of the neocortex. Annual Review of Cell and Developmental Biology. 2014; **30**:465-502

[44] Apple DM, Fonseca RS, Kokovay E. The role of adult neurogenesis in psychiatric and cognitive disorders. Brain Research. 2017;**1655**:270-276

[45] Mu Y, Lee SW, Gage FH. Signaling in adult neurogenesis. Current Opinion in Neurobiology. 2010;**20**(4):416-423

[46] Braun SM, Jessberger S. Adult neurogenesis: Mechanisms and functional significance. Development. 2014;**141**(10):1983-1986

[47] Cameron HA, Glover LR. Adult neurogenesis: Beyond learning and

memory. Annual Review of Psychology. 2015;**66**:53-81

[48] Gage FH. Mammalian neural stem cells. Science. 2000;**287**(5457): 1433-1438

[49] Zhao C, Teng EM, Summers RG, Ming G-l, Gage FH. Distinct morphological stages of dentate granule neuron maturation in the adult mouse hippocampus. Journal of Neuroscience. 2006;**26**(1):3-11

[50] Kempermann G, Jessberger S, Steiner B, Kronenberg G. Milestones of neuronal development in the adult hippocampus. Trends in Neurosciences. 2004;**27**(8):447-452

[51] Toni N, Laplagne DA, Zhao C, Lombardi G, Ribak CE, Gage FH, et al. Neurons born in the adult dentate gyrus form functional synapses with target cells. Nature Neuroscience. 2008; **11**(8):901-907

[52] Aimone JB, Jessberger S, Gage FH. Adult neurogenesis. Scholarpedia. 2007;**2**(2):2100

[53] Ge S, Goh EL, Sailor KA, Kitabatake Y, Ming GL, Song H. GABA regulates synaptic integration of newly generated neurons in the adult brain. Nature. 2006;**439**(7076):589-593

[54] Ge S, Sailor KA, Gl M, Song H. Synaptic integration and plasticity of new neurons in the adult hippocampus. The Journal of Physiology. 2008;**586**(16):3759-3765

[55] Schmidt-Hieber C, Jonas P, Bischofberger J. Enhanced synaptic plasticity in newly generated granule cells of the adult hippocampus. Nature. 2004;**429**(6988):184-187

[56] Alonso M, Viollet C, Gabellec M-M, Meas-Yedid V, Olivo-Marin J-C, Lledo P-M. Olfactory discrimination learning increases the survival of adult-born neurons in the olfactory bulb. Journal of Neuroscience. 2006;**26**(41):10508-10513

[57] Gould E, Beylin A, Tanapat P, Reeves A, Shors TJ. Learning enhances adult neurogenesis in the hippocampal formation. Nature Neuroscience. 1999;**2**(3):260-265

[58] Lugert S, Basak O, Knuckles P, Haussler U, Fabel K, Götz M, et al. Quiescent and active hippocampal neural stem cells with distinct morphologies respond selectively to physiological and pathological stimuli and aging. Cell Stem Cell. 2010;**6**(5): 445-456

[59] Murphy T, Dias GP, Thuret S. Effects of diet on brain plasticity in animal and human studies: Mind the gap. Neural Plasticity. 2014:1-32

[60] Van Riel D, Verdijk R, Kuiken T. The olfactory nerve: A shortcut for influenza and other viral diseases into the central nervous system. The Journal of Pathology. 2015;**235**(2):277-287

[61] Butowt R, Bilinska K. SARS-CoV-2: Olfaction, brain infection, and the urgent need for clinical samples allowing earlier virus detection. ACS Chemical Neuroscience. 2020;**11**(9): 1200-1203

[62] Sungnak W, Huang N, Bécavin C, Berg M, Queen R, Litvinukova M, et al. SARS-CoV-2 entry factors are highly expressed in nasal epithelial cells together with innate immune genes. Nature Medicine. 2020;**26**(5):681-687

[63] Bohmwald K, Gálvez N, Ríos M, Kalergis A. Neurologic alterations due to respiratory virus infections. Frontiers in Cellular Neuroscience. 2018;**12**(386): 2018

[64] Meinhardt J, Radke J, Dittmayer C, Franz J, Thomas C, Mothes R, et al. Olfactory transmucosal SARS-CoV-2 invasion as a port of central nervous

system entry in individuals with COVID-19. Nature Neuroscience. 2021;**24**(2):168-175

[65] Li YC, Bai WZ, Hashikawa T. The neuroinvasive potential of SARS-CoV2 may play a role in the respiratory failure of COVID-19 patients. Journal of Medical Virology. 2020;**92**(6):552-555

[66] Shi Y, Li Z, Yang C, Liu C. The role of gut-brain axis in SARA-CoV-2 neuroinvasion: Culprit or innocent bystander? Brain, Behavior, and Immunity. 2021;**94**:476-477

[67] Desforges M, Le Coupanec A, Dubeau P, Bourgouin A, Lajoie L, Dubé M, et al. Human coronaviruses and other respiratory viruses: Underestimated opportunistic pathogens of the central nervous system? Viruses. 2020;**12**(1):14

[68] Finsterer J, Stollberger C. Update on the neurology of COVID-19. Journal of Medical Virology. 2020;**92**(11): 2316-2318

[69] Li H, Xue Q, Xu X. Involvement of the nervous system in SARS-CoV-2 infection. Neurotoxicity Research. 2020;**1**:1-7

[70] Rabiee A, Nikayin S, Hashem MD, Huang M, Dinglas VD, Bienvenu OJ, et al. Depressive symptoms after critical illness: A systematic review and meta-analysis. Critical Care Medicine. 2016;**44**(9):1744

[71] Nikayin S, Rabiee A, Hashem MD, Huang M, Bienvenu OJ, Turnbull AE, et al. Anxiety symptoms in survivors of critical illness: A systematic review and meta-analysis. General Hospital Psychiatry. 2016;**43**:23-29

[72] Parker AM, Sricharoenchai T, Raparla S, Schneck KW, Bienvenu OJ, Needham DM. Posttraumatic stress disorder in critical illness survivors: A metaanalysis. Critical Care Medicine. 2015;**43**(5):1121-1129

[73] Hopkins RO, Weaver LK, Pope D, Orme JF Jr, Bigler ED, Larson-Lohr V. Neuropsychological sequelae and impaired health status in survivors of severe acute respiratory distress syndrome. American Journal of Respiratory and Critical Care Medicine. 1999;**160**(1):50-56

[74] DeCarolis NA, Eisch AJ. Hippocampal neurogenesis as a target for the treatment of mental illness: A critical evaluation. Neuropharmacology. 2010;**58**(6):884-893

[75] Lu Y, Li X, Geng D, Mei N, Wu P-Y, Huang C-C, et al. Cerebral micro-structural changes in COVID-19 patients–an MRI-based 3-month follow-up study. EClinicalMedicine. 2020;**25**:100484

[76] Gellrich J, Han P, Manesse C, Betz A, Junghanns A, Raue C, et al. Brain volume changes in hyposmic patients before and after olfactory training. The Laryngoscope. 2018;**128**(7):1531-1536

[77] Karstensen HG, Vestergaard M, Baaré WF, Skimminge A, Djurhuus B, Ellefsen B, et al. Congenital olfactory impairment is linked to cortical changes in prefrontal and limbic brain regions. Brain Imaging and Behavior. 2018;**12**(6):1569-1582

[78] Recinto P, Samant ARH, Chavez G, Kim A, Yuan CJ, Soleiman M, et al. Levels of neural progenitors in the hippocampus predict memory impairment and relapse to drug seeking as a function of excessive methamphetamine self-administration. Neuropsychopharmacology. 2012;**37**(5):1275-1287

[79] Misane I, Kruis A, Pieneman AW, Ögren SO, Stiedl O. GABAA receptor activation in the CA1 area of the dorsal hippocampus impairs consolidation of conditioned contextual fear in C57BL/6J mice. Behavioural Brain Research. 2013;**238**:160-169

[80] Aziz M, Goyal H, Haghbin H, Lee-Smith WM, Gajendran M, Perisetti A. The association of "loss of smell" to COVID-19: A systematic review and meta-analysis. The American Journal of the Medical Sciences. 2020;**361**(2):216-225

[81] Meng X, Deng Y, Dai Z, Meng Z. COVID-19 and anosmia: A review based on up-to-date knowledge. American Journal of Otolaryngology. 2020;**41**(5): 102581

[82] Boesveldt S, Postma EM, Boak D, Welge-Luessen A, Schöpf V, Mainland JD, et al. Anosmia—a clinical review. Chemical Senses. 2017;**42**(7): 513-523

[83] Lledo P-M, Valley M. Adult olfactory bulb neurogenesis. Cold Spring Harbor Perspectives in Biology. 2016;**8**(8): a018945

[84] Chiu A, Fischbein N, Wintermark M, Zaharchuk G, Yun PT, Zeineh M. COVID-19-induced anosmia associated with olfactory bulb atrophy. Neuroradiology. 2021;**63**(1):147-148

[85] Galougahi MK, Ghorbani J, Bakhshayeshkaram M, Naeini AS, Haseli S. Olfactory bulb magnetic resonance imaging in SARS-CoV-2-induced anosmia: The first report. Academic Radiology. 2020;**27**(6): 892-893

[86] Sulzer D, Antonini A, Leta V, Nordvig A, Smeyne RJ, Goldman JE, et al. COVID-19 and possible links with Parkinson's disease and parkinsonism: From bench to bedside. npj. Parkinson's Disease. 2020;**6**(1):1-10

[87] Brundin P, Nath A, Beckham JD. Is COVID-19 a perfect storm for Parkinson's disease? Trends in Neurosciences. 2020;**43**(12):931-933

[88] Marxreiter F, Regensburger M, Winkler J. Adult neurogenesis in Parkinson's disease. Cellular and Molecular Life Sciences. 2013;**70**(3): 459-473

[89] Winner B, Kohl Z, Gage FH. Neurodegenerative disease and adult neurogenesis. European Journal of Neuroscience. 2011;**33**(6):1139-1151

[90] Kase Y, Okano H. Expression of ACE2 and a viral virulence-regulating factor CCN family member 1 in human iPSC-derived neural cells: Implications for COVID-19-related CNS disorders. Inflammation and Regeneration. 2020;**40**(1):1-8

[91] Liu S, Liu J, Miura Y, Tanabe C, Maeda T, Terayama Y, et al. Conversion of Aβ43 to Aβ40 by the successive action of angiotensin-converting enzyme 2 and angiotensin-converting enzyme. Journal of Neuroscience Research. 2014;**92**(9): 1178-1186

[92] Kamel AS, Abdelkader NF, Abd El-Rahman SS, Emara M, Zaki HF, Khattab MM. Stimulation of ACE2/ANG[1-7]/Mas axis by diminazene ameliorates Alzheimer's disease in the D-Galactose-ovariectomized rat model: Role of PI3K/Akt pathway. Molecular Neurobiology. 2018;**55**(10):8188-8202

[93] Wang X-L, Iwanami J, Min L-J, Tsukuda K, Nakaoka H, Bai H-Y, et al. Deficiency of angiotensin-converting enzyme 2 causes deterioration of cognitive function. NPJ Aging and Mechanisms of Disease. 2016;**2**(1):1-8

[94] Klempin F, Mosienko V, Matthes S, Villela DC, Todiras M, Penninger JM, et al. Depletion of angiotensin-converting enzyme 2 reduces brain serotonin and impairs the running-induced neurogenic response. Cellular and Molecular Life Sciences. 2018;**75**(19):3625-3634

[95] Hashimoto T, Perlot T, Rehman A, Trichereau J, Ishiguro H, Paolino M, et al. ACE2 links amino acid malnutrition to microbial ecology and

intestinal inflammation. Nature. 2012;**487**(7408):477-481

[96] Chen Y, Chen L, Deng Q, Zhang G, Wu K, Ni L, et al. The presence of SARS-CoV-2 RNA in the feces of COVID-19 patients. Journal of Medical Virology. 2020;**92**(7):833-840

[97] Liang W, Feng Z, Rao S, Xiao C, Xue X, Lin Z, et al. Diarrhoea may be underestimated: A missing link in 2019 novel coronavirus. Gut. 2020;**69**(6): 1141-1143

[98] Viana SD, Nunes S, Reis F. ACE2 imbalance as a key player for the poor outcomes in COVID-19 patients with age-related comorbidities - Role of gut microbiota dysbiosis. Ageing Research Reviews. 2020;**62**:101123

[99] Möhle L, Mattei D, Heimesaat Markus M, Bereswill S, Fischer A, Alutis M, et al. Ly6Chi monocytes provide a link between antibiotic-induced changes in Gut Microbiota and adult hippocampal neurogenesis. Cell Reports. 2016;**15**(9):1945-1956

[100] Peirce JM, Alviña K. The role of inflammation and the gut microbiome in depression and anxiety. Journal of Neuroscience Research. 2019;**97**(10):1223-1241

[101] Koo JW, Duman RS. IL-1β is an essential mediator of the antineurogenic and anhedonic effects of stress. Proceedings of the National Academy of Sciences. 2008;**105**(2):751-756

[102] Borsini A, Alboni S, Horowitz MA, Tojo LM, Cannazza G, Su K-P, et al. Rescue of IL-1β-induced reduction of human neurogenesis by omega-3 fatty acids and antidepressants. Brain, Behavior, and Immunity. 2017; **65**:230-238

[103] Borsini A, Cattaneo A, Malpighi C, Thuret S, Harrison NA, Consortium MI, et al. Interferon-alpha reduces human hippocampal neurogenesis and increases apoptosis via activation of distinct STAT1-dependent mechanisms. International Journal of Neuropsychopharmacology. 2018;**21**(2):187-200

[104] Kempuraj D, Selvakumar GP, Ahmed ME, Raikwar SP, Thangavel R, Khan A, et al. COVID-19, mast cells, cytokine storm, psychological stress, and neuroinflammation. The Neuroscientist. 2020;**26**(5-6):402-414

[105] Pedersen SF, Ho Y-C. SARS-CoV-2: A storm is raging. The Journal of Clinical Investigation. 2020;**130**(5): 2202-2205

[106] Vardhana SA, Wolchok JD. The many faces of the anti-COVID immune response. Journal of Experimental Medicine. 2020;**217**(6):1-10

[107] Hagg T. From neurotransmitters to neurotrophic factors to neurogenesis. The Neuroscientist. 2009;**15**(1):20-27

[108] Walther D, Peter JU, Bashammakh S, Hortnagl H, Voits M, Fink H, et al. Synthesis of serotonin by a second tryptophan hydroxylase isoform. Science. 2003;**299**:76

[109] Malberg JE, Eisch AJ, Nestler EJ, Duman RS. Chronic antidepressant treatment increases neurogenesis in adult rat Hippocampus. The Journal of Neuroscience. 2000;**20**(24):9104-9110

[110] Yan W, Wilson CC, Haring JH. 5-HT1a receptors mediate the neurotrophic effect of serotonin on developing dentate granule cells. Developmental Brain Research. 1997;**98**(2):185-190

[111] Santarelli L, Saxe M, Gross C, Surget A, Battaglia F, Dulawa S, et al. Requirement of hippocampal neurogenesis for the behavioral effects of antidepressants. Science. 2003; **301**(5634):805-809

[112] Banasr M, Hery M, Printemps R, Daszuta A. Serotonin-induced increases in adult cell proliferation and neurogenesis are mediated through different and common 5-HT receptor subtypes in the dentate gyrus and the subventricular zone. Neuropsychopharmacology. 2004; **29**(3):450-460

[113] Brezun J, Daszuta A. Serotonergic reinnervation reverses lesion-induced decreases in PSA-NCAM labeling and proliferation of hippocampal cells in adult rats. Hippocampus. 2000; **10**(1):37-46

[114] Malberg JE, Duman RS. Cell proliferation in adult hippocampus is decreased by inescapable stress: Reversal by fluoxetine treatment. Neuropsychopharmacology. 2003;**28**(9):1562-1571

[115] Jayakumar S, Raghunath G, Ilango S, Vijayakumar J, Vijayaraghavan R. Effect of fluoxetine on the Hippocampus of Wistar Albino rats in cold restraint stress model. Journal of Clinical and Diagnostic Research. 2017;**11**(6):AF01-AAF6

[116] Wang J-W, David DJ, Monckton JE, Battaglia F, Hen R. Chronic fluoxetine stimulates maturation and synaptic plasticity of adult-born hippocampal granule cells. Journal of Neuroscience. 2008;**28**(6):1374-1384

[117] Singer D, Camargo SM, Ramadan T, Schäfer M, Mariotta L, Herzog B, et al. Defective intestinal amino acid absorption in Ace2 null mice. American Journal of Physiology-Gastrointestinal and Liver Physiology. 2012;**303**(6):G686-GG95

[118] Takamura N, Nakagawa S, Masuda T, Boku S, Kato A, Song N, et al. The effect of dopamine on adult hippocampal neurogenesis. Progress in Neuro-Psychopharmacology and Biological Psychiatry. 2014;**50**: 116-124

[119] Winner B, Desplats P, Hagl C, Klucken J, Aigner R, Ploetz S, et al. Dopamine receptor activation promotes adult neurogenesis in an acute Parkinson model. Experimental Neurology. 2009;**219**(2):543-552

[120] Curtis MA, Low VF, Faull RL. Neurogenesis and progenitor cells in the adult human brain: A comparison between hippocampal and subventricular progenitor proliferation. Developmental Neurobiology. 2012;**72**(7):990-1005

[121] Diaz J, Ridray S, Mignon V, Griffon N, Schwartz J-C, Sokoloff P. Selective expression of dopamine D3 receptor mRNA in proliferative zones during embryonic development of the rat brain. Journal of Neuroscience. 1997;**17**(11):4282-4292

[122] Khaindrava V, Salin P, Melon C, Ugrumov M, Kerkerian-Le-Goff L, Daszuta A. High frequency stimulation of the subthalamic nucleus impacts adult neurogenesis in a rat model of Parkinson's disease. Neurobiology of Disease. 2011;**42**(3):284-291

[123] Höglinger GU, Rizk P, Muriel MP, Duyckaerts C, Oertel WH, Caille I, et al. Dopamine depletion impairs precursor cell proliferation in Parkinson disease. Nature Neuroscience. 2004;**7**(7): 726-735

[124] Borta A, Höglinger GU. Dopamine and adult neurogenesis. Journal of Neurochemistry. 2007;**100**(3):587-595

[125] Villar-Cheda B, Dominguez-Meijide A, Valenzuela R, Granado N, Moratalla R, Labandeira-Garcia JL. Aging-related dysregulation of dopamine and angiotensin receptor interaction. Neurobiology of Aging. 2014;**35**(7):1726-1738

[126] Nataf S. An alteration of the dopamine synthetic pathway is possibly involved in the pathophysiology of

COVID-19. Journal of Medical Virology. 2020;**92**(10):1743-1744

[127] Pawlak R, Napiorkowska-Pawlak D, Takada Y, Urano T, Nagai N, Ihara H, et al. The differential effect of angiotensin II and angiotensin 1-7 on norepinephrine, epinephrine, and dopamine concentrations in rat hypothalamus: The involvement of angiotensin receptors. Brain Research Bulletin. 2001;**54**(6):689-694

[128] Merello M, Bhatia KP, Obeso JA. SARS-CoV-2 and the risk of Parkinson's disease: Facts and fantasy. The Lancet Neurology. 2021;**20**(2):94-95

[129] Antonini A, Leta V, Teo J, Chaudhuri KR. Outcome of Parkinson's disease patients affected by COVID-19. Movement Disorders. 2020;**35**(6): 905-908

[130] Rodriguez-Perez AI, Garrido-Gil P, Pedrosa MA, Garcia-Garrote M, Valenzuela R, Navarro G, et al. Angiotensin type 2 receptors: Role in aging and neuroinflammation in the substantia nigra. Brain, Behavior, and Immunity. 2020;**87**:256-271

[131] Loy R, Milner TA. Sexual dimorphism in extent of axonal sprouting in rat hippocampus. Science. 1980;**208**(4449):1282-1284

[132] Jhaveri DJ, Mackay EW, Hamlin AS, Marathe SV, Nandam LS, Vaidya VA, et al. Norepinephrine directly activates adult hippocampal precursors via β3-adrenergic receptors. Journal of Neuroscience. 2010;**30**(7): 2795-2806

[133] Masuda T, Nakagawa S, Boku S, Nishikawa H, Takamura N, Kato A, et al. Noradrenaline increases neural precursor cells derived from adult rat dentate gyrus through beta2 receptor. Progress in Neuro-Psychopharmacology and Biological Psychiatry. 2012;**36**(1): 44-51

[134] Kulkarni VA, Jha S, Vaidya VA. Depletion of norepinephrine decreases the proliferation, but does not influence the survival and differentiation, of granule cell progenitors in the adult rat hippocampus. European Journal of Neuroscience. 2002;**16**(10):2008-2012

[135] Miranda-Contreras L, Ramırez-Martens L, Benítez-Diaz P, Pena-Contreras Z, Mendoza-Briceno R, Palacios-Prü E. Levels of amino acid neurotransmitters during mouse olfactory bulb neurogenesis and in histotypic olfactory bulb cultures. International Journal of Developmental Neuroscience. 2000;**18**(1):83-91

[136] Bolteus AJ, Garganta C, Bordey A. Assays for measuring extracellular GABA levels and cell migration rate in acute slices. Brain Research Protocols. 2005;**14**(2):126-134

[137] Castiglione M, Calafiore M, Costa L, Sortino MA, Nicoletti F, Copani A. Group I metabotropic glutamate receptors control proliferation, survival and differentiation of cultured neural progenitor cells isolated from the subventricular zone of adult mice. Neuropharmacology. 2008;**55**(4): 560-567

[138] Platel J-C, Dave KA, Gordon V, Lacar B, Rubio ME, Bordey A. NMDA receptors activated by subventricular zone astrocytic glutamate are critical for neuroblast survival prior to entering a synaptic network. Neuron. 2010;**65**(6):859-872

[139] Erlander MG, Tillakaratne NJ, Feldblum S, Patel N, Tobin AJ. Two genes encode distinct glutamate decarboxylases. Neuron. 1991;**7**(1):91-100

[140] Cryan JF, Slattery DA. GABAB receptors and depression: Current status. Advances in Pharmacology. 2010;**58**:427-451

[141] Zhu L, Polley N, Mathews GC, Delpire E. NKCC1 and KCC2 prevent hyperexcitability in the mouse hippocampus. Epilepsy Research. 2008;**79**(2-3):201-212

[142] Chancey JH, Adlaf EW, Sapp MC, Pugh PC, Wadiche JI, Overstreet-Wadiche LS. GABA depolarization is required for experience-dependent synapse unsilencing in adult-born neurons. Journal of Neuroscience. 2013;**33**(15): 6614-6622

[143] Liu X, Wang Q, Haydar TF, Bordey A. Nonsynaptic GABA signaling in postnatal subventricular zone controls proliferation of GFAP-expressing progenitors. Nature Neuroscience. 2005;**8**(9):1179-1187

[144] Nguyen L, Malgrange B, Breuskin I, Bettendorff L, Moonen G, Belachew S, et al. Autocrine/paracrine activation of the GABAA receptor inhibits the proliferation of neurogenic polysialylated neural cell adhesion molecule-positive [PSA-NCAM+] precursor cells from postnatal striatum. Journal of Neuroscience. 2003;**23**(8):3278-3294

[145] Bolteus AJ, Bordey A. GABA release and uptake regulate neuronal precursor migration in the postnatal subventricular zone. Journal of Neuroscience. 2004;**24**(35):7623-7631

[146] Tozuka Y, Fukuda S, Namba T, Seki T, Hisatsune T. GABAergic excitation promotes neuronal differentiation in adult hippocampal progenitor cells. Neuron. 2005;**47**(6): 803-815

[147] Nakamichi N, Takarada T, Yoneda Y. Neurogenesis mediated by γ-aminobutyric acid and glutamate signaling. Journal of Pharmacological Sciences. 2009;**110**(2):133-149

[148] Chen R, Wang K, Yu J, Howard D, French L, Chen Z, et al. The spatial and cell-type distribution of SARS-CoV-2 receptor ACE2 in the human and mouse brains. Frontiers in Neurology. 2021; **11**(1860):1-12

[149] Ramani A, Müller L, Ostermann PN, Gabriel E, Abida-Islam P, Müller-Schiffmann A, et al. SARS-CoV-2 targets neurons of 3D human brain organoids. The EMBO Journal. 2020;**39**(20):e106230

[150] Galic MA, Riazi K, Pittman QJ. Cytokines and brain excitability. Frontiers in Neuroendocrinology. 2012;**33**(1):116-125

[151] Nikbakht F, Mohammadkhanizadeh A, Mohammadi E. How does the COVID-19 cause seizure and epilepsy in patients? The potential mechanisms. Multiple Sclerosis and Related Disorders. 2020;**46**:102535

Chapter 2

Neuroimmunology and Neurological Manifestations of COVID-19

Robert Weissert

Abstract

Infection with SARS-CoV-2 is causing coronavirus disease in 2019 (COVID-19). Besides respiratory symptoms due to an attack on the broncho-alveolar system, COVID-19, among others, can be accompanied by neurological symptoms because of the affection of the nervous system. These can be caused by intrusion by SARS-CoV-2 of the central nervous system (CNS) and peripheral nervous system (PNS) and direct infection of local cells. In addition, neurological deterioration mediated by molecular mimicry to virus antigens or bystander activation in the context of immunological anti-virus defense can lead to tissue damage in the CNS and PNS. In addition, cytokine storm caused by SARS-CoV-2 infection in COVID-19 can lead to nervous system related symptoms. Endotheliitis of CNS vessels can lead to vessel occlusion and stroke. COVID-19 can also result in cerebral hemorrhage and sinus thrombosis possibly related to changes in clotting behavior. Vaccination is most important to prevent COVID-19 in the nervous system. There are symptomatic or/and curative therapeutic approaches to combat COVID-19 related nervous system damage that are partly still under study.

Keywords: SARS-CoV-2, COVID-19, CNS, PNS, T cell, B cell, vaccination, treatment, neuroimmunology, molecular mimicry, bystander activation, cytokine storm

1. Introduction

Severe acute respiratory syndrome coronavirus 2 (SARS-CoV-2) is a single-stranded positive sense ribonucleic acid (ssRNA) virus with an envelope that leads to coronavirus disease 2019 (COVID-19) [1]. COVID-19 has affected millions of people worldwide since its emergence in December 2019 in Wuhan in China. It has caused a worldwide pandemic. Multiple mutated variants of SARS-CoV-2 have appeared with varying infectivity [2, 3]. SARS-CoV-2 has caused major disease burden and death rates worldwide. Due to the threat to individual health and health systems, SARS-CoV-2 and COVID-19 have resulted in a worldwide social and economic crisis. Economically rich Western countries have success in fighting SARS-CoV-2 by vaccination, while this is not true to the same extent for economically weak countries due to a shortage of vaccine supply. In addition, the standard of care for patients with COVID-19 differs dramatically based on the economic wealth of a country [4]. Due to the nature of the pandemic to affect people worldwide, there is a lack of help from rich countries for economically weak countries.

2. Background

SARS-CoV-2 is a beta-coronavirus [5]. The positive ssRNA genome encodes 16 non-structural proteins involved in viral replication. Moreover, four structural proteins are for the envelope, spike-glycoprotein, the membrane, and the nucleocapsid [6]. Angiotensin-converting enzyme 2 (ACE2) is the receptor for uptake of SARS-CoV-2 [7–9]. Co-factors are heparan sulfates on the cell surface [10]. The spike protein is of major importance for interaction with ACE2 and cellular uptake. ACE2 is expressed in many cells of the body and therefore SARS-CoV-2 can infect most organs. SARS-CoV-2 uses the infected cell for the production of the virus. More receptors and host factors have been described for SARS-CoV-2 cellular entry [11, 12]. Most cells in the body express ACE2 receptors mediating SARS-CoV-2 uptake.

SARS-CoV-2 has the strongest effects on the lung [13, 14]. As a result of infection, SARS-CoV-2 leads to an atypical mainly interstitial pneumonia with patchy infiltrates. In severe cases, the lung can be completely affected resulting in loss of oxygenation. Besides the lung, any tissue can be infected by SARS-CoV-2 and damaged. As written further down and explained for the nervous system, the tissue damage can be a consequence of direct infection with the virus or indirect effects on the tissue due to a dysregulated immune response.

3. Hypoxia and CNS damage

Reduced oxygenation caused by SARS-CoV-2 mediated pneumonia in COVID-19 can lead to severe hypoxia of CNS. In many cases of patients that have died of COVID-19, severe hypoxia of the CNS has been observed [15]. There is an acute hypoxic-ischemic injury with neuronal loss and the presence of apoptotic neurons. This kind of CNS damage is unrelated to direct viral infection of the CNS or indirect effects mediated by the virus-induced immune response within the CNS but a consequence of the strongly reduced oxygenation of erythrocytes in the lung. This reduced oxygenation of erythrocytes results in hypoxia of the CNS. Besides hypoxia, at biopsy or autopsy in CNS microthrombi, thromboembolic disease, inflammation, and to the largest extent hemodynamic mediated changes were found [16].

4. Direct effects of SARS-CoV-2 in CNS

There is evidence that SARS-CoV-2 can be present in CNS [17–19]. There are indications that SARS-CoV-2 can infect many CNS-resident cells [20, 21]. The presence of SARS-CoV-2 in cells is causing cellular dysfunction resulting in a variety of manifestations [22]. For example, infection of olfactory bulb neurons with SARS-CoV-2 will lead to olfactory dysfunction (dysosmia). In addition, infection of neurons involved in taste sensing will lead to the reduction of taste perception (ageusia). Dysosmia and ageusia have been observed early on in patients with COVID-19 [23]. Subsequently, evidence for direct infection of other parts of the CNS has been found (**Table 1**).

5. Vasculature and COVID-19

SARS-CoV-2 infection can lead to endotheliitis [36, 40]. Endotheliitis, caused by SARS-CoV-2 infection also affect CNS vessels. In endotheliitis, there is an

Disease manifestation	Structure	Diagnostics	Treatment
Dysosmia [23, 24]	Olfactory bulb	C.e., NMR, odor testing	None
Ageusia [23, 24]	Gustatory neurons	C.e., NMR, taste testing	None
Decreased cognitive function [25]	Hippocampus	C.e., cCT, cNMR, neuropsychological testing	None
Encephalitis [26]	Brain parenchyma	C.e., cCT, cNMR, CSF, EEG	If present, treatment of cerebral edema; treatment of co-infections
Meningitis [27, 28]	Meninges	C.e., cCT, cNMR, CSF	If present, treatment of cerebral edema; treatment of co-infections
Headache [29]	Meninges and brain parenchyma	C.e., CT, NMR, CSF	If present, treatment of cerebral edema
Dizziness [30]	Brain parenchyma, occlusive vessel disease	C.e., cCT, cNMR, CSF	Antiplatelet therapy, statin
Impaired consciousness [31]	Brain parenchyma, occlusive vessel disease	C.e., cCT, cNMR, CSF	If present, treatment of cerebral edema; treatment of infections; if occlusive vessel disease antiplatelet therapy, statin
Epileptic seizures [32, 33]	Brain parenchyma	C.e., EEG, cCT, cNMR, CSF	Antiepileptics
Cerebral ischemia [34, 35]	Occlusive vessel disease, thromboembolism	C.e., cCT, cNMR, ultrasound	Antiplatelet therapy, statin
Cerebral bleeding [36]	Angiitis	C.e., cCT, cNMR, CSF	Depending on severity, neurosurgical intervention
Cerebral venous thrombosis [37]	Changes in blood clotting behavior	C.e., cCT, cNMR, CSF	Aspirin or anticoagulation depending on severity
Posterior reversible encephalopathy [38, 39]	Unknown	C.e., cCT, cNMR, CSF, EEG	None

c, cerebral; C.e., clinical examination; CNS, central nervous system; CSF, cerebrospinal-fluid; CT, computer tomography; EEG, electroencephalography; NMR, nuclear magnetic resonance.

Table 1.
Manifestations of putative direct infection of cells with consequences in the CNS in COVID-19.

accumulation of lymphocytes, neutrophils, and macrophages in endothelial walls. Endotheliitis can have major consequences eventually resulting in ischemic stroke. Also, alternative mechanisms of damage to large and small cerebral vessels by SARS-CoV-2 in COVID-19 have been observed [41]. In the heart, it has been shown that endotheliitis leads to small vessel vasculitis. This can also involve epicardial nerves in COVID-19 disease with the appearance of an inflammatory neuropathy, possibly resulting in cardiac complications such as myocardial injury and arrhythmias [42].

6. Indirect effects of SARS-CoV-2 in CNS

There are several neurological symptoms and diseases that are associated with COVID-19. These include Guillain-Barré-syndrome (GBS), myasthenia gravis (MG), opsoclonus-myoclonus syndrome (OMS) and others (**Table 2**). In these diseases, a direct effect of SARS-CoV-2 and subsequent tissue damage is unlikely and other mechanisms are hypothesized. Such potential mechanisms are molecular mimicry and bystander activation [61, 62]. Molecular mimicry means that there may be the structural similarity between virus sequences or/and domains and structures or/and sequences of the individual [63]. Potentially, these similarities can result in an immune response that is not only directed against parts of the virus but also against self-proteins, for example, the nicotinic acetylcholine receptor (nAChR) that is the autoantigen in myasthenia gravis. In bystander activation, the immune response triggered by a viral infection can cause an activation of an immune response directed against self-antigens that will also result in autoimmune disease. The list of possible autoimmune manifestations due to the affection of SARS-CoV-2 and COVID-19 is growing. This is also the case for autoimmune neurological manifestations (**Table 2**). There is increasing knowledge regarding the structural requirements for induction of autoimmune disease after viral infection with SARS-CoV-2.

Cytokine storm induced by infection with SARS-CoV-2 and COVID-19 can lead to multiple organ damage and potentially induction/boosting of an autoimmune immune response [54].

7. Chronic fatigue syndrome and COVID-19

Some patients that had COVID-19 subsequently develop long-COVID-19 or also named post-COVID-19 [64, 65]. Many of these patients suffer from strong fatigue. The condition is clinically like chronic fatigue syndrome (CFS) also named myalgic encephalomyelitis (ME). In CFS there is a strong indication that there is an energy failure on the cellular level that can result in rapid exhaustion and fatigue. In addition, there are changes in certain immune cell types that can result in increased susceptibility to infection. Changes in lymphocyte stiffness, monocyte size, neutrophil size and deformability, and heterogeneity of erythrocyte deformation and size were found [66]. The exact mechanism of how COVID-19 is resulting in subsequent CFS is not known at present. The diagnosis is mainly based on clinical characteristics with the presence of abnormal fatigue. Presently, there are no specific markers that allow a laboratory-based diagnosis. Usually, CSF analysis does not show distinctive features. There are no approved pharmaceutical options for the treatment of fatigue associated with long-COVID-19 or post-COVID-19. Treatment involves mild physical endurance training.

8. Treatment of COVID-19

Treatment options can be separated according to treatment to counteract viral replication and viral virulence of SARS-CoV-2 and treatment options to counteract and treat organ damage due to consequences of the infection with SARS-CoV-2 (**Table 3**). Remdesivir is a treatment option that counteracts viral replication [67]. This is a drug that has been initially developed for fighting Ebola. It has been shown to be efficacious if given early after infection with SARS-CoV-2. In combination with the Janus-kinase inhibitor baricitinib increased efficacy could be demonstrated [69].

Disease	Disease mechanism	Autoantigen	Diagnostics	Treatment
Myasthenia gravis [43, 44]	Muscular weakness due to antibodies against proteins of the neuromuscular junction	nAChR, MUSK	C.e., determination of autoantibodies, repetitive nerve stimulation	Acetylcholine esterase inhibitors, steroids, plasmapheresis immunosuppressants/ immunomodulators
Guillain-Barré-syndrome [45, 46]	Demyelination of peripheral nerves due to activation of the adaptive and innate immune system by viral triggers	Schwann-cell-derived proteins	C.e., neurography, CSF	Plasmapheresis, immunoglobulins
Cranial nerve demyelination [47, 48]	Demyelination of cranial nerves due to activation of the adaptive and innate immune system by viral triggers	Cranial nerve proteins	C.e., neurography, CSF, cNMR	Plasmapheresis, immunoglobulins
Opsoclonus-myoclonus syndrome [49]	Rare neuroimmunological disorder with ocular, motor, behavioral, sleep, and language disturbances and ataxia.	Neuronal proteins	C.e., cCT, cNMR, CSF	Steroids, plasmapheresis, immunoglobulins, depletion of B cells
Cerebellar ataxia [50, 51]	Inflammatory disease of the cerebellum with ataxia, vertigo, and visual disturbances	Neuronal proteins	C.e., cCT, cNMR, CSF	Steroids, plasmapheresis, depletion of B cells
Transverse myelitis [52]	Inflammatory disease of the myelon with resulting paresis or paralysis (mono, para, tetra), sensory disturbances, and bladder dysfunction	Oligodendroglial- or astrocytic proteins	C.e., sNMR, cNMR, CSF	Steroids, plasmapheresis, depletion of B cells
Limbic encephalitis, autoimmune encephalitis [53, 54]	Encephalitis with autoimmune pathogenesis	Neuronal proteins	C.e., cNMR, CSF, EEG, neuropsychological testing	Steroids, plasmapheresis, immunoglobulins, depletion of B cells
Multiple sclerosis [55]	Autoimmune disease of CNS resulting in inflammation, demyelination, and axonal loss with a multitude of resulting symptoms	MBP, PLP, and other oligodendrocyte-derived proteins	C.e., cNMR, CSF	Steroids, immunomodulatory treatment
Anti-MOG disease [56]	Autoimmune disease of the CNS with lesion development and resulting neurological symptoms	MOG	C.e., cNMR, CSF	Steroids

Disease	Disease mechanism	Autoantigen	Diagnostics	Treatment
Acute disseminated encephalomyelitis (ADEM) [17, 57]	Inflammatory disease of the CNS with associated neurological symptoms	MBP, others	C.e., cNMR, CSF	Steroids
Acute hemorrhagic leukoencephalitis, acute necrotizing encephalopathy [58]	Severe inflammatory and hemorrhagic disease of the CNS with high neurological disease burden	Cytokine storm [59]	C.e., cCT, cNMR, CSF	Steroids
Bickerstaff's encephalitis [60]	Inflammatory disease of the brain stem with cranial nerve palsies and ataxia	Glial- and neuronal proteins	C.e., cNMR, neurophysiological studies, CSF	Steroids
Generalized myoclonus [51]	Inflammatory disease affecting neuronal structures with resulting myoclonus	Neuronal proteins	C.e., cCT, cNMR, CSF	Steroids, piracetam

c, cerebral; C.e., clinical examination; CSF, cerebro-spinal-fluid; CT, computer tomography; EEG, electroencephalography; MBP, myelin basic protein; MOG, myelin oligodendrocyte glycoprotein; MuSK, muscle-specific tyrosine kinase; nAChR, nicotinic acetylcholine receptor; NMR, nuclear magnetic resonance; PLP, proteolipid protein; sc, spinal cord.

Table 2.
Autoimmune diseases of the nervous system have been reported in the context of COVID-19.

Treatment	Approach	Efficacy
Remdesivir [67, 68]	Inhibition of viral replication	Shortening the time to recovery in adults who were hospitalized with COVID-19 and had evidence of lower respiratory tract infection; in combination with baricitinib superior efficacy. Among nonhospitalized patients who were at high risk for COVID-19 progression, a 3-day course of remdesivir in an 87% lower risk of hospitalization or death than placebo.
Baricitinib [69]	Janus-kinase Inhibitor (JAK1 and JAK2)	Mainly in patients receiving oxygen support without invasive mechanical ventilation.
Dexamethasone [70]	Antiinflammatory	Lower 28-day mortality in hospitalized patients among those who were receiving either invasive mechanical ventilation or oxygen alone at randomization but not among those receiving no respiratory support; increased mortality compared with usual care in patients not requiring oxygen supplementation.
Tocilizumab [71–73]	anti-IL-6R blockade	Reduces the risk of mechanical ventilation in hospitalized patients with severe COVID-19; improved outcome and survival of COVID-19.
Sarilumab [73]	anti-IL-6R blockade	Improved outcome and survival of COVID-19.
Anakinra [74]	anti-IL-1R blockade	Early increase of soluble urokinase plasminogen activator receptor (suPAR) serum was used as a marker to assess the risk of COVID-19. Early start of treatment with anakinra guided by suPAR levels in patients hospitalized with moderate and severe COVID-19 significantly reduced the risk of worse clinical outcome at day 28 and reduced length of hospital stay compared to placebo.
Regdanvimab [75]	Blockade of spike protein interaction with ACE2	Regdanvimab reduced the risk of hospitalization or death versus placebo in patients with mild-to-moderate COVID-19 symptoms who were considered at high risk of progressing to severe COVID-19 up to day 28.
Casirivimab/Imdevimab [76]	Blockade of spike protein interaction with ACE2	Casirivimab/Imdevimab reduced the risk of COVID-19-related hospitalization or death from any cause, and it resolved symptoms and reduced the SARS-CoV-2 viral load more rapidly than placebo.
Sotrovimab [77]	Neutralisation SARS-CoV-2	The risk of disease progression was reduced among high-risk patients with mild-to-moderate COVID-19 treated with sotrovimab.
Molnupiravir [78]	anti-RNA polymerase activity	The risk of hospitalization or death in at-risk, unvaccinated adults with COVID-19 was reduced in patients treated early with molnupiravir.

Treatment	Approach	Efficacy
Tixagevimab/Cilgavimab [79]	Neutralization of SARS-CoV-2	Preliminary results indicate a decrease in disease severity in COVID-19 patients.
PV-07321332/Ritanovir [79]	Protease Inhibitor of SARS-CoV-2 3-chymotrypsin-like protease	Reduction of risk of hospitalization and death compared to placebo in adults with a high risk of poor outcome of COVID-19

ACE, angiotensin-converting enzyme; COVID-19, coronavirus disease 2019; JAK, janus-kinase; IL-1R, interleukin-1 receptor; IL-6R, interleukin-6 receptor.

Table 3.
Treatment options to counteract viral replication or/and viral virulence or organ damage caused by a viral infection or virus-mediated secondary tissue damage.

Dexamethasone has been shown to have beneficial effects in COVID-19 since it leads to reduction of the host immune response against the virus [70]. This host immune response can lead to catastrophic outcomes for the body. Beneficial effects of dexamethasone are mainly seen in the case of severely ill patients requiring mechanical ventilation. In non-severely affected COVID-19 patients not requiring oxygen supplementation, increased mortality is observed [80]. Tocilizumab an anti-interleukin-6 receptor (IL-6R) directed monoclonal antibody (mAb) has been shown to have some beneficial effects in COVID-19 patients reducing the risk of mechanical assistance [71, 72]. Also, another mAb against IL-6R, Sarilumab, improved the outcome and survival of COVID-19 [73]. Early start of treatment with anakinra a mAb against the interleukin-1 receptor (IL-1R) guided by levels against soluble urokinase plasminogen activator receptor (suPAR) significantly reduced the risk of worse clinical outcome at day 28 and reduced the length of hospital stay compared to placebo in patients hospitalized with moderate and severe COVID-19 [74]. Various mAb directed against the SARS-CoV-2 spike protein have demonstrated beneficial effects in patients with COVID-19 [76, 77, 79]. Malnupavir has anti-RNA polymerase activity and the risk of hospitalization or death in at-risk, unvaccinated adults with COVID-19 was reduced in patients treated early with this novel compound [78]. The protease inhibitor PV-07321332/Ritanovir of SARS-COV-2 3-chymotrypsin-like protease resulted in the reduction of risk of hospitalization and death compared to placebo in adults with a high risk of poor outcome of COVID-19 [79]. Much effort is done to identify compounds with beneficial effects in COVID-19 patients including repurposing of drugs from other indications [73, 81]. Importantly, serum from patients recovered from COVID-19 has been used successfully to reduce mortality in patients with active COVID-19 disease [82]. Higher anti-SARS-COV-2 titers of the transfused plasma led to a lower risk of death in non-ventilated patients with COVID-19. So far, besides symptomatic treatments no specific treatments for COVID-19- related neurological conditions have been introduced. Nevertheless, the beneficial effects of treatment on COVID-19 precipitation and severity will also result in reduced neurological disease burden.

9. Vaccination

Vaccination is of paramount importance to counteract the further spreading of SARS-CoV-2 and COVID-19 [83]. The first vaccines were introduced at the end of 2020 [84] and the beginning of 2021 [85–87]. Since then, a major vaccination effort has been undertaken with the fastest vaccination campaigns in Israel and Great Britain. The vaccines also have shown efficacy against mutated variants of SARS-CoV-2 even though breakthrough infections have been observed [88]. Societies with high numbers of vaccinated individuals have gained better control over the COVID-19 pandemic compared to societies with low vaccination rates. Repetitive vaccination strategies have increased vaccination efficacy and have provided more protection from novel virus variants [89]. Presently as of the end of January 2022, mRNA vaccines and adenovirus vectors with inserts of sequences coding for the spike protein of SARS-CoV-2 and protein-based vaccines have been introduced [84–87, 90, 91]. Vaccination efficacy is much dependent on booster vaccination regimes [89, 92, 93]. All currently approved vaccines are given by intramuscular injection [94]. Muscle cells that take up the mRNA vaccine or the adenovirus-vector-based vaccine are used subsequently to produce SARS-CoV-2- derived spike protein. This protein is recognized as `non-self` by the immune system and a strong T-and B-cell derived immune response is generated. This immune response leads to protection from SARS-CoV-2. The protein-based vaccines lead to the generation of a T- and B-cell response against SARS-CoV-2. There are vaccination-related cases with neurological symptoms [95–97]. In general, vaccination-related side effects were increased in patients with preceding COVID-19 [98].

10. Conclusion

Infection with SARS-CoV-2 resulting in COVID-19 leads to damage of many organs in the body. The nervous system is also often assaulted by the virus and the subsequent immune response. The treatment options are limited. Vaccination to prevent the spread of SARS-CoV-2 and its variants is the most efficacious way to prevent nervous system disease in context with SARS-CoV-2 and COVID-19. Possibly, the insights that are obtained on the worldwide population level by SARS-CoV-2 and COVID-19 will result in a better understanding of the induction of autoimmune disease of the nervous system in general.

Conflict of interest

The author declares no conflict of interest.

Author details

Robert Weissert
Department of Neurology, University of Regensburg, Germany

*Address all correspondence to: robert.weissert@googlemail.com or robert.weissert@ukr.de

References

[1] Zhu N, Zhang D, Wang W, Li X, Yang B, Song J, et al. A Novel coronavirus from patients with pneumonia in China, 2019. New England Journal of Medicine. 2020;**382**(8):727-733

[2] Abdool Karim SS, de Oliveira T. New SARS-CoV-2 variants—Clinical, public health, and vaccine implications. New England Journal of Medicine. 2021; **384**(19):1866-1868

[3] Viana R, Moyo S, Amoako DG, Tegally H, Scheepers C, Althaus CL, et al. Rapid epidemic expansion of the SARS-CoV-2 Omicron variant in southern Africa. Nature. 2022 [Online ahead of print]

[4] Oehler RL, Vega VR. Conquering COVID: How global vaccine inequality risks prolonging the pandemic. Open Forum Infectious Diseases. 2021;**8**(10): ofab443

[5] Malik YA. Properties of coronavirus and SARS-CoV-2. Malaysian Journal of Pathology. 2020;**42**(1):3-11

[6] Yao H, Song Y, Chen Y, Wu N, Xu J, Sun C, et al. Molecular architecture of the SARS-CoV-2 virus. Cell. 2020;**183**(3):730-8 e13

[7] Wang Q, Zhang Y, Wu L, Niu S, Song C, Zhang Z, et al. Structural and functional basis of SARS-CoV-2 entry by using human ACE2. Cell. 2020;**181**(4):894-904 e9

[8] Yan R, Zhang Y, Li Y, Xia L, Guo Y, Zhou Q. Structural basis for the recognition of SARS-CoV-2 by full-length human ACE2. Science. 2020;**367**(6485):1444-1448

[9] Zhou P, Yang XL, Wang XG, Hu B, Zhang L, Zhang W, et al. A pneumonia outbreak associated with a new coronavirus of probable bat origin. Nature. 2020;**579**(7798):270-273

[10] Clausen TM, Sandoval DR, Spliid CB, Pihl J, Perrett HR, Painter CD, et al. SARS-CoV-2 infection depends on cellular heparan sulfate and ACE2. Cell. 2020;**183**(4):1043-57 e15

[11] Wei J, Alfajaro MM, DeWeirdt PC, Hanna RE, Lu-Culligan WJ, Cai WL, et al. Genome-wide CRISPR screens reveal host factors critical for SARS-CoV-2 infection. Cell. 2021;**184**(1): 76-91 e13

[12] Wang R, Simoneau CR, Kulsuptrakul J, Bouhaddou M, Travisano KA, Hayashi JM, et al. Genetic screens identify host factors for SARS-CoV-2 and common cold coronaviruses. Cell. 2021;**184**(1): 106-19 e14

[13] Shi H, Han X, Jiang N, Cao Y, Alwalid O, Gu J, et al. Radiological findings from 81 patients with COVID-19 pneumonia in Wuhan, China: A descriptive study. Lancet Infectious Diseases. 2020;**20**(4):425-434

[14] Zhang N, Xu X, Zhou LY, Chen G, Li Y, Yin H, et al. Clinical characteristics and chest CT imaging features of critically ill COVID-19 patients. European Radiology. 2020;**30**(11): 6151-6160

[15] Solomon IH, Normandin E, Bhattacharyya S, Mukerji SS, Keller K, Ali AS, et al. Neuropathological features of Covid-19. New England Journal of Medicine. 2020;**383**(10):989-992

[16] Peiris S, Mesa H, Aysola A, Manivel J, Toledo J, Borges-Sa M, et al. Pathological findings in organs and tissues of patients with COVID-19: A systematic review. PLoS One. 2021;**16**(4):e0250708

[17] Reichard RR, Kashani KB, Boire NA, Constantopoulos E, Guo Y, Lucchinetti CF. Neuropathology of

COVID-19: A spectrum of vascular and acute disseminated encephalomyelitis (ADEM)-like pathology. Acta Neuropathology. 2020;**140**(1):1-6

[18] Matschke J, Lutgehetmann M, Hagel C, Sperhake JP, Schroder AS, Edler C, et al. Neuropathology of patients with COVID-19 in Germany: A post-mortem case series. The Lancet Neurology. 2020;**19**(11):919-929

[19] von Weyhern CH, Kaufmann I, Neff F, Kremer M. Early evidence of pronounced brain involvement in fatal COVID-19 outcomes. Lancet. 2020;**395**(10241):e109

[20] Pajo AT, Espiritu AI, Apor A, Jamora RDG. Neuropathologic findings of patients with COVID-19: A systematic review. Neurological Sciences. 2021;**42**(4):1255-1266

[21] Gagliardi S, Emanuele Poloni T, Pandini C, Garofalo M, Dragoni F, Medici V, et al. Detection of SARS-CoV-2 genome and whole transcriptome sequencing in frontal cortex of COVID-19 patients. Brain, Behavior, and Immunity. 2021;**97**:13-21

[22] Qin Y, Wu J, Chen T, Li J, Zhang G, Wu D, et al. Long-term microstructure and cerebral blood flow changes in patients recovered from COVID-19 without neurological manifestations. Journal of Clinical Investigation. 2021;**131**(8)

[23] Wolfel R, Corman VM, Guggemos W, Seilmaier M, Zange S, Muller MA, et al. Virological assessment of hospitalized patients with COVID-2019. Nature. 2020;**581**(7809):465-469

[24] Lechien JR, Chiesa-Estomba CM, De Siati DR, Horoi M, Le Bon SD, Rodriguez A, et al. Olfactory and gustatory dysfunctions as a clinical presentation of mild-to-moderate forms of the coronavirus disease (COVID-19): A multicenter European study. European Archives of Oto-Rhino-Laryngology. 2020;**277**(8):2251-2261

[25] Alnefeesi Y, Siegel A, Lui LMW, Teopiz KM, Ho RCM, Lee Y, et al. Impact of SARS-CoV-2 infection on cognitive function: A systematic review. Frontiers in Psychiatry. 2020;**11**:621773

[26] Pilotto A, Odolini S, Masciocchi S, Comelli A, Volonghi I, Gazzina S, et al. Steroid-Responsive encephalitis in coronavirus disease 2019. Annals of Neurology. 2020;**88**(2):423-427

[27] Moriguchi T, Harii N, Goto J, Harada D, Sugawara H, Takamino J, et al. A first case of meningitis/encephalitis associated with SARS-Coronavirus-2. International Journal of Infectious Diseases. 2020;**94**:55-58

[28] Khodamoradi Z, Hosseini SA, Gholampoor Saadi MH, Mehrabi Z, Sasani MR, Yaghoubi S. COVID-19 meningitis without pulmonary involvement with positive cerebrospinal fluid PCR. European Journal of Neurology. 2020;**27**(12):2668-2669

[29] Huang C, Wang Y, Li X, Ren L, Zhao J, Hu Y, et al. Clinical features of patients infected with 2019 novel coronavirus in Wuhan, China. Lancet. 2020;**395**(10223):497-506

[30] Wu F, Zhao S, Yu B, Chen YM, Wang W, Song ZG, et al. A new coronavirus associated with human respiratory disease in China. Nature. 2020;**579**(7798):265-269

[31] Kotfis K, Williams Roberson S, Wilson JE, Dabrowski W, Pun BT, Ely EW. COVID-19: ICU delirium management during SARS-CoV-2 pandemic. Critical Care. 2020;**24**(1):176

[32] Lu L, Xiong W, Liu D, Liu J, Yang D, Li N, et al. New onset acute symptomatic seizure and risk factors in coronavirus disease 2019: A

retrospective multicenter study. Epilepsia. 2020;**61**(6):e49-e53

[33] Mithani F, Poursheykhi M, Ma B, Smith RG, Hsu SH, Gotur D. New-onset seizures in three COVID-19 patients: A case series. Journal of Clinical Neurophysiology. 2021;**38**(2):e5-e10

[34] Beyrouti R, Adams ME, Benjamin L, Cohen H, Farmer SF, Goh YY, et al. Characteristics of ischaemic stroke associated with COVID-19. Journal of Neurology, Neurosurgery, and Psychiatry. 2020;**91**(8):889-891

[35] Yaghi S, Ishida K, Torres J, Mac Grory B, Raz E, Humbert K, et al. SARS-CoV-2 and stroke in a New York healthcare system. Stroke. 2020; **51**(7):2002-2011

[36] Kirschenbaum D, Imbach LL, Rushing EJ, Frauenknecht KBM, Gascho D, Ineichen BV, et al. Intracerebral endotheliitis and microbleeds are neuropathological features of COVID-19. Neuropathology and Applied Neurobiology. 2021;**47**(3):454-459

[37] Cavalcanti DD, Raz E, Shapiro M, Dehkharghani S, Yaghi S, Lillemoe K, et al. Cerebral venous thrombosis associated with COVID-19. AJNR. American Journal of Neuroradiology. 2020;**41**(8):1370-1376

[38] Kishfy L, Casasola M, Banankhah P, Parvez A, Jan YJ, Shenoy AM, et al. Posterior reversible encephalopathy syndrome (PRES) as a neurological association in severe Covid-19. Journal of the Neurological Sciences. 2020;**414**:116943

[39] Coolen T, Lolli V, Sadeghi N, Rovai A, Trotta N, Taccone FS, et al. Early postmortem brain MRI findings in COVID-19 non-survivors. Neurology. 2020;**95**(14):e2016-e2e27

[40] Varga Z, Flammer AJ, Steiger P, Haberecker M, Andermatt R, Zinkernagel AS, et al. Endothelial cell infection and endotheliitis in COVID-19. Lancet. 2020;**395**(10234):1417-1418

[41] Keller E, Brandi G, Winklhofer S, Imbach LL, Kirschenbaum D, Frontzek K, et al. Large and small cerebral vessel involvement in severe COVID-19: Detailed clinical workup of a case series. Stroke. 2020;**51**(12): 3719-3722

[42] Maccio U, Zinkernagel AS, Shambat SM, Zeng X, Cathomas G, Ruschitzka F, et al. SARS-CoV-2 leads to a small vessel endotheliitis in the heart. eBioMedicine. 2021;**63**:103182

[43] Huber M, Rogozinski S, Puppe W, Framme C, Hoglinger G, Hufendiek K, et al. Postinfectious onset of Myasthenia Gravis in a COVID-19 patient. Frontiers in Neurology. 2020;**11**:576153

[44] Restivo DA, Centonze D, Alesina A, Marchese-Ragona R. Myasthenia Gravis associated with SARS-CoV-2 infection. Annals of International Medicine. 2020;**173**(12):1027-1028

[45] Zhao H, Shen D, Zhou H, Liu J, Chen S. Guillain-Barre syndrome associated with SARS-CoV-2 infection: Causality or coincidence? Lancet Neurology. 2020;**19**(5):383-384

[46] Toscano G, Palmerini F, Ravaglia S, Ruiz L, Invernizzi P, Cuzzoni MG, et al. Guillain-Barre syndrome associated with SARS-CoV-2. New England Journal of Medicine. 2020;**382**(26):2574-2576

[47] Dinkin M, Gao V, Kahan J, Bobker S, Simonetto M, Wechsler P, et al. COVID-19 presenting with ophthalmoparesis from cranial nerve palsy. Neurology. 2020;**95**(5):221-223

[48] Gutierrez-Ortiz C, Mendez-Guerrero A, Rodrigo-Rey S, San Pedro-Murillo E, Bermejo-Guerrero L, Gordo-Manas R, et al. Miller Fisher syndrome and polyneuritis cranialis in

COVID-19. Neurology. 2020;**95**(5):e601-e6e5

[49] Emamikhah M, Babadi M, Mehrabani M, Jalili M, Pouranian M, Daraie P, et al. Opsoclonus-myoclonus syndrome, a post-infectious neurologic complication of COVID-19: Case series and review of literature. Journal of Neurovirology. 2021;**27**(1):26-34

[50] Werner J, Reichen I, Huber M, Abela IA, Weller M, Jelcic I. Subacute cerebellar ataxia following respiratory symptoms of COVID-19: A case report. BMC Infectious Diseases. 2021;**21**(1):298

[51] Chan JL, Murphy KA, Sarna JR. Myoclonus and cerebellar ataxia associated with COVID-19: A case report and systematic review. Journal of Neurology. 2021;**268**(10):3517-3548

[52] Moreno-Escobar MC, Kataria S, Khan E, Subedi R, Tandon M, Peshwe K, et al. Acute transverse myelitis with dysautonomia following SARS-CoV-2 infection: A case report and review of literature. Journal of Neuroimmunology. 2021;**353**:577523

[53] Pizzanelli C, Milano C, Canovetti S, Tagliaferri E, Turco F, Verdenelli S, et al. Autoimmune limbic encephalitis related to SARS-CoV-2 infection: Case-report and review of the literature. Brain, Behavior, & Immunity-Health. 2021;**12**:100210

[54] Valencia Sanchez C, Theel E, Binnicker M, Toledano M, McKeon A. Autoimmune encephalitis after SARS-CoV-2 infection: Case frequency, findings, and outcomes. Neurology. 2021;**97**(23):e2262-e22e8

[55] Palao M, Fernandez-Diaz E, Gracia-Gil J, Romero-Sanchez CM, Diaz-Maroto I, Segura T. Multiple sclerosis following SARS-CoV-2 infection. Multiple Sclerosis and Related Disorders. 2020;**45**:102377

[56] Jumah M, Rahman F, Figgie M, Prasad A, Zampino A, Fadhil A, et al. COVID-19, HHV6 and MOG antibody: A perfect storm. Journal of Neuroimmunology. 2021;**353**:577521

[57] Shahmirzaei S, Naser MA. Association of COVID-19 and acute disseminated encephalomyelitis (ADEM) in the absence of pulmonary involvement. Autoimmunity Reviews. 2021;**20**(3):102753

[58] Delamarre L, Gollion C, Grouteau G, Rousset D, Jimena G, Roustan J, et al. COVID-19-associated acute necrotising encephalopathy successfully treated with steroids and polyvalent immunoglobulin with unusual IgG targeting the cerebral fibre network. Journal of Neurology, Neurosurgery, and Psychiatry. 2020;**91**(9):1004-1006

[59] Bhaskar S, Sinha A, Banach M, Mittoo S, Weissert R, Kass JS, et al. Cytokine storm in COVID-19-immunopathological mechanisms, clinical considerations, and therapeutic approaches: The REPROGRAM consortium position paper. Frontiers in Immunology. 2020;**11**:1648

[60] Llorente Ayuso L, Torres Rubio P, Beijinho do Rosario RF, Giganto Arroyo ML, Sierra-Hidalgo F. Bickerstaff encephalitis after COVID-19. Journal of Neurology. 2020;**268**(6):2035-2037

[61] Guadarrama-Ortiz P, Choreno-Parra JA, Sanchez-Martinez CM, Pacheco-Sanchez FJ, Rodriguez-Nava AI, Garcia-Quintero G. Neurological aspects of SARS-CoV-2 infection: Mechanisms and manifestations. Frontiers in Neurology. 2020;**11**:1039

[62] Riedhammer C, Weissert R. Antigen presentation, autoantigens, and immune regulation in multiple sclerosis and

other autoimmune diseases. Frontiers in Immunology. 2015;**6**:322

[63] Khamsi R. Rogue antibodies could be driving severe COVID-19. Nature. 2021;**590**(7844):29-31

[64] Yong SJ. Long COVID or post-COVID-19 syndrome: Putative pathophysiology, risk factors, and treatments. Infectious Diseases. 2021;**1-18**

[65] Salamanna F, Veronesi F, Martini L, Landini MP, Fini M. Post-COVID-19 Syndrome: The persistent symptoms at the post-viral stage of the disease. A systematic review of the current data. Frontiers in Medicine. 2021;**8**:653516

[66] Kubankova M, Hohberger B, Hoffmanns J, Furst J, Herrmann M, Guck J, et al. Physical phenotype of blood cells is altered in COVID-19. Biophysics Journal. 2021;**120**(14): 2838-2847

[67] Beigel JH, Tomashek KM, Dodd LE. Remdesivir for the treatment of Covid-19—Preliminary report reply. New England Journal of Medicine. 2020;**383**(10):994

[68] Gottlieb RL, Vaca CE, Paredes R, Mera J, Webb BJ, Perez G, et al. Early remdesivir to prevent progression to severe Covid-19 in outpatients. New England Journal of Medicine. 2022;**386**(4):305-315

[69] Kalil AC, Patterson TF, Mehta AK, Tomashek KM, Wolfe CR, Ghazaryan V, et al. Baricitinib plus remdesivir for hospitalized adults with Covid-19. New England Journal of Medicine. 2021;**384**(9):795-807

[70] Group RC, Horby P, Lim WS, Emberson JR, Mafham M, Bell JL, et al. Dexamethasone in hospitalized patients with Covid-19. New England Journal of Medicine. 2021;**384**(8):693-704

[71] Rosas IO, Brau N, Waters M, Go RC, Hunter BD, Bhagani S, et al. Tocilizumab in hospitalized patients with severe Covid-19 pneumonia. New England Journal of Medicine. 2021;**384**(16):1503-1516

[72] Salama C, Han J, Yau L, Reiss WG, Kramer B, Neidhart JD, et al. Tocilizumab in patients hospitalized with Covid-19 pneumonia. New England Journal of Medicine. 2021;**384**(1):20-30

[73] Investigators R-C, Gordon AC, Mouncey PR, Al-Beidh F, Rowan KM, Nichol AD, et al. Interleukin-6 receptor antagonists in critically Ill patients with Covid-19. New England Journal of Medicine. 2021;**384**(16):1491-1502

[74] Kyriazopoulou E, Poulakou G, Milionis H, Metallidis S, Adamis G, Tsiakos K, et al. Early treatment of COVID-19 with anakinra guided by soluble urokinase plasminogen receptor plasma levels: a double-blind, randomized controlled phase 3 trial. Nature Medicine. 2021;**27**(10):1752-1760

[75] Syed YY. Regdanvimab: First approval. Drugs. 2021;**81**(18):2133-2137

[76] Weinreich DM, Sivapalasingam S, Norton T, Ali S, Gao H, Bhore R, et al. REGEN-COV antibody combination and outcomes in outpatients with covid-19. New England Journal of Medicine. 2021;**385**(23):e81

[77] Gupta A, Gonzalez-Rojas Y, Juarez E, Crespo Casal M, Moya J, Falci DR, et al. Early treatment for Covid-19 with SARS-CoV-2 neutralizing antibody sotrovimab. New England Journal of Medicine. 2021;**385**(21): 1941-1950

[78] Jayk Bernal A, Gomes da Silva MM, Musungaie DB, Kovalchuk E, Gonzalez A, Delos Reyes V, et al. Molnupiravir for oral treatment of Covid-19 in nonhospitalized patients.

New England Journal of Medicine. 2022;**386**(6):509-520

[79] Garcia-Lledo A, Gomez-Pavon J, Gonzalez Del Castillo J, Hernandez-Sampelayo T, Martin-Delgado MC, Martin Sanchez FJ, et al. Pharmacological treatment of COVID-19: An opinion paper. Revista Española de Quimioterapia. 2021 [Online ahead of print]

[80] Johns M, George S, Taburyanskaya M, Poon YK. A review of the evidence for corticosteroids in COVID-19. Journal of Pharmacy Practice. 2021 897190021998502

[81] Consortium WHOST, Pan H, Peto R, Henao-Restrepo AM, Preziosi MP, Sathiyamoorthy V, et al. Repurposed antiviral drugs for Covid-19—Interim WHO solidarity trial results. New England Journal of Medicine. 2021;**384**(6):497-511

[82] Joyner MJ, Carter RE, Senefeld JW, Klassen SA, Mills JR, Johnson PW, et al. Convalescent plasma antibody levels and the risk of death from Covid-19. New England Journal of Medicine. 2021;**384**(11):1015-1027

[83] Amanat F, Krammer F. SARS-CoV-2 vaccines: Status report. Immunity. 2020;**52**(4):583-589

[84] Polack FP, Thomas SJ, Kitchin N, Absalon J, Gurtman A, Lockhart S, et al. Safety and efficacy of the BNT162b2 mRNA Covid-19 vaccine. New England Journal of Medicine. 2020;**383**(27): 2603-2615

[85] Baden LR, El Sahly HM, Essink B, Kotloff K, Frey S, Novak R, et al. Efficacy and safety of the mRNA-1273 SARS-CoV-2 vaccine. New England Journal of Medicine. 2021;**384**(5): 403-416

[86] Voysey M, Clemens SAC, Madhi SA, Weckx LY, Folegatti PM, Aley PK, et al. Safety and efficacy of the ChAdOx1 nCoV-19 vaccine (AZD1222) against SARS-CoV-2: An interim analysis of four randomised controlled trials in Brazil, South Africa, and the UK. Lancet. 2021;**397**(10269):99-111

[87] Sadoff J, Gray G, Vandebosch A, Cardenas V, Shukarev G, Grinsztejn B, et al. Safety and efficacy of single-dose Ad26.COV2.S vaccine against Covid-19. New England Journal of Medicine. 2021;**384**(10):2187-2201

[88] Hacisuleyman E, Hale C, Saito Y, Blachere NE, Bergh M, Conlon EG, et al. Vaccine breakthrough infections with SARS-CoV-2 variants. New England Journal of Medicine. 2021;**384**(23): 2212-2218

[89] Sablerolles RSG, Rietdijk WJR, Goorhuis A, Postma DF, Visser LG, Geers D, et al. Immunogenicity and reactogenicity of vaccine boosters after Ad26.COV2.S priming. New England Journal of Medicine. 2022 [Online ahead of print]

[90] Dunkle LM, Kotloff KL, Gay CL, Anez G, Adelglass JM, Barrat Hernandez AQ, et al. Efficacy and safety of NVX-CoV2373 in adults in the United States and Mexico. New England Journal of Medicine. 2022;**386**(6):531-543

[91] Voysey M, Costa Clemens SA, Madhi SA, Weckx LY, Folegatti PM, Aley PK, et al. Single-dose administration and the influence of the timing of the booster dose on immunogenicity and efficacy of ChAdOx1 nCoV-19 (AZD1222) vaccine: A pooled analysis of four randomised trials. Lancet. 2021;**397**(10277):881-891

[92] Bar-On YM, Goldberg Y, Mandel M, Bodenheimer O, Freedman L, Kalkstein N, et al. Protection of BNT162b2 vaccine booster against Covid-19 in Israel. New England Journal of Medicine. 2021;**385**(15):1393-1400

[93] Nemet I, Kliker L, Lustig Y, Zuckerman N, Erster O, Cohen C, et al. Third BNT162b2 vaccination neutralization of SARS-CoV-2 omicron infection. New England Journal of Medicine. 2022;**386**(5):492-494

[94] Garcia-Montero C, Fraile-Martinez O, Bravo C, Torres-Carranza D, Sanchez-Trujillo L, Gomez-Lahoz AM, et al. An updated review of SARS-CoV-2 vaccines and the importance of effective vaccination programs in pandemic times. Vaccine. 2021;**9**(5)

[95] Perry RJ, Tamborska A, Singh B, Craven B, Marigold R, Arthur-Farraj P, et al. Cerebral venous thrombosis after vaccination against COVID-19 in the UK: A multicentre cohort study. Lancet. 2021;**398**(10306):1147-1156

[96] Schulz JB, Berlit P, Diener HC, Gerloff C, Greinacher A, Klein C, et al. COVID-19 vaccine-associated cerebral venous thrombosis in Germany. Annals of Neurology. 2021;**90**(4):627-639

[97] Havla J, Schultz Y, Zimmermann H, Hohlfeld R, Danek A, Kumpfel T. First manifestation of multiple sclerosis after immunization with the Pfizer-BioNTech COVID-19 vaccine. Journal of Neurology. 2022;**269**(1):55-58

[98] Barda N, Dagan N, Ben-Shlomo Y, Kepten E, Waxman J, Ohana R, et al. Safety of the BNT162b2 mRNA Covid-19 vaccine in a nationwide setting. New England Journal of Medicine. 2021;**385**(12):1078-1090

Chapter 3

COVID-19 and Seizures

Rafael Jesus, Carolina Azoia, Paulo Coelho and Pedro Guimarães

Abstract

The past two years were deeply marked by the emergence of a global pandemic caused by the worldwide spread of the virus *severe acute respiratory syndrome coronavirus type 2* (SARS-CoV-2) infection. The plethora of repercussions on the health of those affected is extensive, ranging from asymptomatic individuals, mild flu-like disease, and severe respiratory failure, eventually leading to death. Despite this predilection for the respiratory system, the virus is responsible for multisystemic manifestations and soon became clear that neurological involvement was a frequent issue of *coronavirus disease 2019* (COVID-19). Much have been pointed out about the neurotropic nature of the virus, the ways by which it invades and targets specific structures of the central nervous system, and the physiopathology behind the neurologic manifestations associated with it (namely encephalomyelitis, Guillain-Barré syndrome, lacunar infarcts, and vascular dysfunction, just to list a few). This chapter aims to raise light about the association between COVID-19 and the mechanisms of acute symptomatic seizures, through neurotropism and neuroinvasion features of SARS-CoV-2, and to review the variety of clinical presentations reported so far.

Keywords: COVID-19, neurotropism, central nervous system infection, acute symptomatic seizure, electroencephalogram

1. Introduction

When SARS-CoV-2 emerged in a seafood wholesale market in Wuhan, a city in the Hubei Province of China, back in December 2019, the world was far from foreseeing the real dimensions of the challenge ahead. What was first considered as just a local outbreak causing a cluster of cases of a "deadly viral pneumonia," soon became a global concern as it spread throughout the five continents in a matter of few months. While reaching pandemic proportions, in 2020, it revealed to have catastrophic healthcare and socioeconomic effects, being responsible for more than 3 million of confirmed cases worldwide and over 200.000 deaths, all in less than six months. The actual number of infections led to more than 299 million cases and over 5.4 million deaths worldwide (data from Johns Hopkins University Coronavirus Resource Center).

SARS-CoV-2 belongs to the family *Coronaviridae*, a large family of viruses that cause illness ranging from the common cold to more severe diseases [1]. Coronaviruses are enveloped positive-stranded RNA viruses, with crown-like thorns on their surface (the Latin word for crown is *coronam*); full-genome sequencing and phylogenic analysis indicate that SARS-CoV-2 is a betacoronavirus in the same subgenus as its older relative SARS-CoV, both distantly related with the *Middle East respiratory syndrome* (MERS) virus [2, 3]. The analysis of the SARS-CoV-2 genome suggests that a natural evolutionary process between a bat-CoV and a pangolin-CoV could have been important in creating the new zoonotic virus, but the closest RNA sequence similarity is to bat coronaviruses, making bats the most probable primary source of human transmission [1, 4]. SARS-CoV-2 enters host cells via the angiotensin-converting enzyme 2 (ACE2) receptor, which is widely expressed in various human organs, particularly in neurons and glia, and to which it binds through the receptor-binding domain of its spike protein [1, 5].

According to the World Health Organization, COVID-19 symptoms can be divided in *most common*, *less common,* and *serious* [6]. Most common symptoms include fever, cough, tiredness, and loss of taste or smell. Less common symptoms include sore throat, headache, generalized aches and pains, diarrhea, rash, and even red, irritated eyes. When it comes to serious symptoms, these include shortness of breath, chest pain, and some neurologic complications such as loss of speech or mobility and confusion. Gladly, the majority of infected people will develop mild to moderate illness and recover without hospitalization; for those who experience severe manifestations, big effort is put on preventing lethal respiratory failure [6].

Recent reports have drawn attention to the neurotropic behavior shown by the virus, as it affects both the central and the peripheral nervous system (CNS and PNS, respectively), as well as skeletal muscle [7]. The neurological diseases affecting the PNS and muscle in COVID-19 are less frequent than those related to the CNS invasion by the virus and include Guillain-Barré syndrome; Miller Fisher syndrome; multiple cranial neuropathies; and rare instances of viral myopathy with rhabdomyolysis [7].

Most frequently described CNS manifestations include headache and agitation, delirium, impaired consciousness, anosmia, hyposmia, hypogeusia, and dysgeusia, some of which are early symptoms of coronavirus infection [7]. Even the respiratory infection has a probable neurogenic origin and may result from the viral invasion of the olfactory nerve, progressing into rhinencephalon and brainstem respiratory centers [7]. Cerebrovascular disease seems to be due to a prothrombotic state induced by viral attachment to ACE2 receptors in endothelium, causing widespread endotheliitis, coagulopathy, arterial and venous thrombosis; acute hemorrhagic necrotizing encephalopathy has also been documented secondary to the cytokine storm involved in the immune response against the virus [7].

To date, literature is still very scarce when it comes to reports of encephalopathy, meningitis, encephalitis, myelitis, and seizures. Given the already proven neurotropism as a common feature of coronaviruses, it is reasonable to expect that some patients infected with SARS-CoV-2 develop seizures as a consequence of hypoxia, metabolic derangements, organ failure, or even cerebral damage that may occur in the context of COVID-19 [8]. This chapter focuses on the specific matter of acute symptomatic seizures associated with COVID-19 with particular interest in the neurologic mechanisms explaining the epileptogenic activity of SARS-CoV-2.

2. About neurotropism: how SARS-CoV-2 affects nervous system

As soon as the scientific community became aware of the multitude and magnitude of neurological complications of SARS-CoV-2 infection, as well as of the fact that virus is detectable in the cerebrospinal fluid (CSF) of patients infected, much effort was put on finding out the many possible ways the virus can enter and affect the nervous system, for a better understanding of pathophysiology and possible treatment targets [9].

Nervous system invasion has already been demonstrated as a feature of previously identified human coronavirus (namely MERS-CoV and SARS-CoV) [10], but it is not clear yet whether neurological symptoms are a direct result of virus infection of nervous system cells, parainfectious or postinfectious immune-related disease, or a consequence of systemic illness, with possible concurring mechanisms [11].

There have been described two different ways for the virus to reach the central nervous system: using a hematogenous route or by a retrograde axonal route. In the hematogenous route, virus circulating in blood vessels gains access to the CNS through infection of endothelial cells at the blood–brain barrier (BBB), epithelial cells at the choroid plexus and immune cells that eventually enter the CNS (the so called "Trojan horse" method). In the retrograde axonal route, the virus travels backward through the axons to reach neuron cell bodies in the peripheral nervous system or in the CNS through neural-mucosal interface [9, 12].

Several ways have been proposed by which SARS-CoV-2 originates neurological damage, including direct damage through receptors in neurons and glia, or indirectly *via* systemic inflammation with cytokine-mediated injury, secondary hypoxia, and retrograde travel through nerve fibers [9].

2.1 The role of angiotensin-converting enzyme 2 (ACE2)

Early in the pandemic, several studies identified ACE2 expressing cells as targets for SARS-CoV-2 infection. Superficial ACE2 works as a functional receptor for the virus to enter into host cells, similarly as for the previously known SARS-CoV, but with higher binding affinity [12, 13].

ACE2 is a carboxy-peptidase responsible for the synthesis of vasodilator peptides as angiotensin-(1-7) [12] and is widely expressed in almost all human organs in varying degrees. It is present in the brain tissue (both neuronal and glial cells) and endothelial cells of BBB allowing viral binding and entry into CNS [5].

Thereby, in the beginning, it was assumed by some authors that ACE2 deficiency could reduce the impact of SARS-CoV-2 infection [14]. Further studies rejected this hypothesis as they concluded that the interaction between ACE2 and SARS-CoV-2 ultimately leads to substantial loss of ACE2 receptor activity on membrane surface, mainly through its internalization, downregulation, and malfunction. Consequently, there is dysregulation of the protective renin-angiotensin-aldosterone system axis inducing higher levels of angiotensin II and less generation of (protective) angiotensin-(1-7). This gives rise to angiotensin II "storm" triggering vasoconstriction and inflammation, kidney failure, heart disease, apoptosis, and oxidative processes that promote brain degeneration and contribute to the poor outcome seen in many patients with COVID-19 and giving rise to some neurological complications [15, 16].

The binding of SARS-CoV-2 with ACE2 receptor gained more significance in cerebrovascular disease in COVID-19 patients as the imbalance of renin-angiotensin-aldosterone axis results in vascular dysfunction leading to atherosclerosis, arterial hypertension, and cardiovascular disease. Along with the prothrombotic effect of inflammatory cascade, it contributes to a higher risk for stroke and venous thrombosis in these patients [12, 15, 17].

2.2 Neuronal retrograde dissemination and neural-mucosal interface

Hyposmia and dysgeusia soon started to be widely reported in patients with SARS-COV-2 infection. One study with 417 patients with mild to moderate COVID-19 found olfactory and gustatory dysfunction in 85,6% and 88% of patients, respectively [18]. These symptoms do not seem to be related to traditional nasal symptoms, as seen in other viral infections (as influenza and rhinovirus), as COVID-19 patients do not present significant nasal congestion or rhinorrhea [15]. Therefore, scientific community postulated that anosmia and dysgeusia could be a consequence of viral infection targeting olfactory system. Further studies suggested that SARS-CoV-2 could directly affect the olfactory nerve and bulb and trigeminal afferents in nasal mucosa and vagus nerve afferents in the respiratory tract, traveling retrogradely along these structures, being a highway between the nasal epithelium and central nervous system [9, 12, 15, 19]. One study assessed viral load of olfactory mucosa and its nervous projections as several other CNS regions in postmortem COVID-19 patients. Higher levels of viral RNA for SARS-CoV-2 were found within the olfactory mucosa directly beneath the cribriform plate, but also in lower levels in the cornea, conjunctiva, and oral mucosa, pointing these as potential sites for SARS-CoV-2 CNS entry. Virus detection in CNS regions with no direct connection to the olfactory mucosa suggests the contribution of other mechanisms in combination with axonal transport, as SARS-CoV-2-containing-leukocyte migrating across the BBB and viral entry along CNS endothelia [19].

Against this theory, some authors showed two important genes for SARS-CoV-2 cellular entry, ACE2 and transmembrane serine protease 2 (TMPRSS2), which were expressed in the olfactory and nasal airway epithelial cells, but not in olfactory afferent neurons, raising questions about the olfactory bulb as a pathway for CNS invasion by SARS-CoV-2 [20]. Frequent and early alterations of taste and smell in patients with COVID-19 reinforce the contribution of a neural-mucosal interface possibly relating to other molecular ways than ACE2 receptor [9, 19].

2.3 Systemic inflammatory response and hypoxia

Neuronal damage can be either the result of viral replication effects or the aberrant immunological response, consequently giving rise to neurological signs and symptoms [12].

The binding of SARS-CoV-2 to pulmonary epithelial cells gives rise to a systemic inflammatory response (SIRS), mediated by increased levels of interleukin (IL), namely IL-6, IL-12, IL-15, and tumor necrosis factor alpha (TNF-α), the so-called "cytokine storm" [9, 21]. The infiltrated immune cells, which include activated astrocytes and microglia, produce even more inflammatory mediators (including cytokines and matrix metalloproteases) resulting in severe brain inflammation. Besides the chemokine role in host defense, they also are responsible for immune damage by attracting activated T cells, NK cells, and monocytes to the brain tissue. TNF-α and Monocyte Chemoattractant Protein-1 (MCP-1) contribute to disruption of tight junctions of the BBB, increasing vascular permeability and leukocyte migration [12, 22], and all this inflammatory cascade causes even more damage to BBB facilitating SARS-CoV-2 invasion of brain cells [10, 15, 22].

Some authors defend that SARS-CoV-2 has antigenic determinants similar to some of myelinated neurons, and a cross-reaction of immunological response to the virus could lead to a postinfectious autoimmune demyelinating disease as encephalomyelitis or acute demyelinating polyneuropathy [22, 23].

Additionally to the systemic inflammatory response, diffuse alveolar and interstitial inflammatory exudation leads to disruption of alveolar gas exchange causing hypoxia in the CNS. This process can also complicate with hemodynamic changes leading to septic (distributive) shock and CNS hypoperfusion. Consequently, this increases anaerobic metabolism in the brain cells with accumulation of acid metabolites that lead to vasodilation, brain edema, and possibly obstruction of blood flow with consequent hypoxic and ischemic lesions of brain tissue [9, 10].

3. SARS-CoV-2 infection and acute symptomatic seizures

Seizure is a relatively uncommon neurological complication of SARS-CoV-2 infection, accounting for less than 1% of patients [17, 24, 25], despite a significant proportion of patients presenting risk factors such as hypoxia, acute cerebrovascular disease, and metabolic derangements [26]. Prevalence was lower compared with previous MERS-CoV and SARS-CoV (8,6% and 2,7%, respectively) [24, 27].

Acute symptomatic seizures can occur in infection setting particularly in patients with poor general condition and fever [25], but a few case reports stated it as a presenting symptom of SARS-CoV-2 infection without the classical respiratory symptoms [27–29]. No study has yet clarified any direct relation between COVID-19 and the potentiation of epileptic seizures. At least in some patients with a history of epilepsy, they could merely reflect unprovoked seizures [26].

Nonetheless, several mechanisms were proposed for seizure generation and epileptogenesis in SARS-CoV-2 infection setting.

3.1 Pro-convulsant effect of angiotensin II

Some reports suggested that ACE2 could also be part of a specific mechanism for seizure induction by SARS-CoV-2, with upregulation of components of the renin-angiotensin-aldosterone in the hippocampus of patients with temporal lobe epilepsy. Downregulation of ACE2 would lead to higher concentration of angiotensin II with angiotensin II receptor type 1 (AT1) activation, which is known to cause vasoconstriction and promote inflammatory cascade. ACE2 also plays a role in kallikrein-kinin system, important for maintenance of cardiovascular system homeostasis. These findings point to a pro-convulsant effect of angiotensin II, theoretically increasing susceptibility to seizure occurrence in COVID-19. However, no experimental or clinical data have yet supported this hypothesis yet [26].

3.2 Neuroinflammation and BBB dysfunction

CSF SARS-CoV-2 PCR was reported positive in some patients with clinical and imagiological evidence of encephalitis. This suggests that the virus is able to invade and infect CNS, causing meningitis and encephalitis with possible concurrent seizures [15]. Neuroinflammation may also be acquired from systemic circulation through BBB dysfunction [30, 31]. Glial cells assume an important role in this process by releasing inflammatory mediators and by modulating neuronal function. Seizure generation and epileptogenesis have been associated with neuronal damage and gliosis and, for some time, with an inflammatory state in neural tissue [30].

After CNS invasion, SARS-CoV-2 triggers a large inflammatory cycle that leads to chronic inflammation and neural hyperexcitability, promoting neuronal apoptosis, astrogliosis, and tissue necrosis [32]. There are several proinflammatory cytokines involved in this process, namely IL-1β, TNF-α, IL-6, but also nitric oxide, prostaglandin-E2 (PGE2), and free radicals. IL-1β, expressed in active microglia and astrocytes, increases availability of glutamate in the synapses and increases the number of GluN2B subunits in NMDA receptors of postsynaptic cells leading to hyperexcitability and possibly causing seizures [30, 32]. TNF-α also plays a role in lowering seizure threshold through induction of glutamate release from glia, increasing excitatory glutamate receptors, and decreasing the number of inhibitory GABA receptors and hyperregulating AMPA receptors (leading to calcium over-uptake and neuronal toxicity) [30, 32]. IL-6 is typically found in low amounts in the CNS, but its levels increase with activation of astrocytes and microglia. This upregulation decreases hippocampal neurogenesis and contributes to initiation of epileptogenesis. PGE2 stimulates EP3 receptors on astrocytes also promoting glutamate release and neuronal hyperexcitability and death [30]. In response to neuronal depolarization and upregulation of these proinflammatory cytokines, matrix metalloproteinase-9 (MMP-9) transcription increases. MMP-9 is responsible for structural modification in synapses, reducing its plasticity, increasing susceptibility to seizure occurrence and epileptogenesis [30, 33]. Chemokines, expressed by microglia, astrocytes, and endothelial cells, can also modify neuronal physiology, modulating ion channels and promoting the release of certain neurotransmitters, contributing to the ictal phenomena [30].

Central and peripheral inflammation and hypoxia contribute to BBB breakdown and dysfunction, through upregulation of inflammatory mediators [31]. Similar to other infectious diseases, COVID-19 infection can affect BBB integrity. This leads to migration of blood cells and proteins and to expression of adherence molecules allowing immune cells to enter [30, 32]. Leucocytes also secrete MMP-9 with the subsequent upregulation of inflammatory mediators, which enhance BBB dysfunction, recruit even more immune cells and astrocyte, and activate glia cells, perpetuating a chronic inflammatory process. The ultimate consequence of this cascade of events is the disruption of osmotic balance in CNS leading to neuronal damage, alteration of membrane potential, hyperexcitable status, and seizure genesis [32].

Hyperthermia is another cause of BBB disruption and a potential seizure inducer. In the brain, severe hyperthermia promotes glial cells activation and increases BBB permeability, *per se*, and indirectly through the release of inflammatory mediators (as IL-1β) [32].

Several studies show that “cytokine storm” and systemic inflammation are responsible for severe cases of acute respiratory distress syndrome and multiorganic failure [34, 35]. Neuroinflammation seems to be a crucial mechanism for seizure occurrence and epileptogenesis in COVID-19 patients [30].

In patients with epilepsy history, infections (mainly respiratory) are a frequent precipitant of relapsing seizures, particularly in pediatric setting [27].

3.3 Metabolic and electrolytic imbalance, hypoxia, and organ failure

Acute symptomatic seizures can occur in patients with metabolic derangements, as the result of COVID-19 multiorganic dysfunction or aggravation of previous comorbidities.

Several works reported metabolic and electrolytic abnormalities in patients with COVID-19, mainly in those patients with severe disease. The most common disorders are decreased serum concentrations of sodium, potassium, calcium, and magnesium, but the pathophysiology is not well elucidated [36, 37]. Some authors propose hypokalemia could result from elevated angiotensin II levels and consequent promotion of renal potassium excretion. Other potential causes for electrolyte imbalance are renal failure, syndrome of inappropriate anti-diuretic hormone secretion (SiADH), iatrogenic (as use of diuretics) and gastrointestinal losses when vomiting and diarrhea are present [36]. Electrolyte disturbances are important causes of acute symptomatic seizures, mainly in patients with hyponatremia, hypocalcaemia, and hypomagnesemia. The successful treatment of these patients is achieved through a correct diagnosis of underlying disturbance and the respective correction, preventing inadequate use of anti-seizure drugs [32, 38].

COVID-19 can also influence glucose metabolism predisposing to higher risk of ketoacidosis in diabetic patients [39]. Even though nonketotic hyperosmolar coma more commonly results in seizures than ketoacidosis, this is a hypothesis to consider in these patients [40].

Systemic inflammatory cascade with endothelial dysfunction and increased brain vasculature permeability and edema can originate a form of posterior reversible encephalopathy syndrome (PRES) concurring as another mechanism for seizure generation. Hypertension and renal disease are predisposing factors for PRES, aggravated by COVID-19 [41].

Severe respiratory disease results in devastating hypoxia that can potentiate hypoxic encephalopathy and contribute to development of seizures. Multiorganic failure as systemic complication of COVID-19 with associated metabolic disorders (namely uremia and metabolic acidosis) could also lead to seizure occurrence [42]. These situations reduce the seizure threshold mostly in susceptible patients (with brain structural lesions or neurodegenerative diseases, for example), potentially causing new-onset seizures or decompensating disease control in patients with previous epilepsy [32].

3.4 Hypercoagulability and cerebrovascular disease

Coagulation disorders and cerebrovascular disease were described soon in a significant number of COVID-19 patients [15]. COVID-19 patients have shown increased levels of D-dimers, which is thought to be associated to the hypercoagulable state and predisposition to thrombosis [22]. One study found much higher rates of diffuse intravascular coagulation in non-survivors compared with survivors, setting that coagulopathy is related to worst prognosis [43, 44]. Different factors can contribute to coagulation disorders. Persistent inflammatory and "cytokine storm" status activates coagulation cascade and suppresses the fibrinolytic system. The resulting endothelial damage by direct effect of the virus (remember ACE2 is expressed in endothelial cells) [22] and aggravated by systemic inflammatory response can activate coagulation system. On the other hand, coagulation cascade can potentiate immune response giving rise to a vicious cycle that progressively increases hypercoagulable state [32, 43].

Thereby, cerebrovascular disease, mainly ischemic events, is a serious complication of COVID-19, occurring in 1–3% of infections (with higher incidence in severe infection setting) [9, 24, 45]. It seems to be the result of hypercoagulable state, direct endothelial damage by SARS-CoV-2, higher levels of angiotensin II associated vasoconstriction, and higher vascular resistance and multiorganic dysfunction that often lead to cardiac malfunction and hypotension, promoting brain ischemia and hypoxia [15, 22].

A seizure can occur as a manifestation of stroke setting with several contributing factors that include hypoxia, metabolic disorders, and imbalance of blood perfusion. In the acute ischemia, damaged cells release potassium and glutamate into the extracellular space, which may activate AMPA and NMDA receptors potentiating neuronal death and contributing for seizure occurrence. Chronic inflammation, gliosis, and neuronal death with alteration of synapses structure and loss of synaptic plasticity contribute to occurrence of late seizures, as well [32, 46].

3.5 Role of mitochondrial dysfunction

Mitochondria play a key role, not only in assuring energy homeostasis, but also in calcium homeostasis, production of reactive oxygen species (ROS), modulation of neurotransmitters in CNS, and regulation of cell apoptosis [47].

COVID-19 infection is associated with oxidative stress, as inflammatory cascade increases production of ROS. High concentrations of ROS can damage mitochondrial respiratory chain, alteration of its membrane permeability and its structure and induce mitochondrial DNA mutations. Due to the important role of these organelles in maintaining normal electrical activity of neuronal and synaptic transmission, any disturbance may lead to abnormal electrical activity of neurons and occurrence of seizures [32, 47].

3.6 Iatrogenic induced seizures

Iatrogenics is another way by which SARS-CoV-2 can be related to acute symptomatic seizures in the context of COVID-19. Drugs used to treat infection—namely chloroquine and hydroxychloroquine—may cause seizures, along with headache, lightheadedness, and paresthesia; liponavir-ritonavir may also cause peripheral and perioral paresthesia, headache, confusion, and reduction of the epileptic threshold [48].

Certain antibiotics were also associated with acute symptomatic seizures. Despite COVID-19 being a viral infection, some patients can evolve with bacterial superinfection and initiate treatment with antibiotics that predispose for seizures, as it is the case for quinolones [49].

4. Clinical features of seizures associated with COVID-19

As mentioned above, in addition to respiratory symptoms, COVID-19 has been associated with neurologic complications, but minimal literature exists about seizures in these patients [50]. Seizures have been described as direct consequence of SARS-CoV infection in the context of encephalitis [51] or indirectly as a consequence of hypoxemia, metabolic derangement, medications, multiorganic failure, or even brain damage [52]. The evidence available points to the fact that the virus by itself does not carry an increased risk of seizure [50], and it is common to find accompanying seizure-triggering comorbidities in patients with a first seizure and COVID-19, mainly metabolic and electrolytic disturbances and ischemic stroke [27].

New-onset seizures in COVID-19 patients should be considered acute symptomatic, and long-term anti-seizure medication is usually not necessary, unless a subsequent episode occurs or a brain lesion is found to raise the risk for seizure recurrence [53].

COVID-19 may present in many different ways making early diagnosis difficult and delaying proper treatment in atypical cases [27]. Even though seizures are not a common manifestation of COVID-19, they have been described in a variety of forms, as focal motor, generalized motor, convulsive and nonconvulsive status epilepticus (CSE and NCSE, respectively) [52]. In most cases, they are not the presenting symptom and arise mostly in patients with severe disease [26].

New-onset seizures had been described as a possible early symptom of COVID-19 in patients with no preceding symptoms suggestive of that diagnosis and, in some cases, seizure is in fact the symptom that prompts presentation to the emergency room, mainly in children [27]. Fasano and colleagues [28] reported a case of first motor seizure as presenting symptom of SARS-CoV-2 infection; Kadono and coworkers [54] described a case of a patient presenting an acute symptomatic seizure with a recurrence of severe brain edema post cerebral venous thrombosis who was later found to have a COVID-19 infection.

Change in mental status has been reported in about 10% of patients with severe COVID-19, but **electroencephalogram** (EEG) has not been done as routine to investigate or exclude NCSE in patients with altered responsiveness and COVID-19 [4, 53]. Several studies report that, due to the contagious nature of the disease, COVID-19 patients had limited access to diagnostic investigations, including EEG, and this could seriously underestimate the incidence of non-motor seizures and NCSE [55].

According to semiology, CSE predominates over NCSE [56]. Nonetheless, COVID-19 patients with unexplained altered mental status should be studied for the possibility of NCSE [42]. Some authors recommend continuous EEG monitoring in patients with COVID-19 and altered mental status to rule out NCSE [8].

5. Complementary studies in SARS-CoV-2 infected patients with seizures

5.1 CSF findings

There are only a few reports with CSF findings in COVID-19 patients, as it is not systematically accessed for every patient. One systematic review reported CSF findings in COVID-19 patients who presented seizures in infection setting, including 69 patients. They found that only 13% had positive CSF SARS-CoV-2 PCR. Pleocytosis was found in one-third of them, and nearly half had increased proteinorachia. Postictal pleocytosis and hyperproteinorachia were already described, so these findings may be secondary to seizures itself as opposed to an intrathecal process related to SARS-CoV-2. Autoimmune antibodies were tested in 11 patients and were positive in only two (NMDA antibodies and Caspr2 antibodies). It remained unclear if these findings were related to COVID-19 (as some cases of autoimmune encephalitis can be preceded by infection that works as a trigger of autoimmunity) or if it was purely coincidental [57].

5.2 Electroencephalographic findings

There are some reports of electroencephalogram (EEG) findings in patients with SARS-CoV-2 infection. Altered mental status and seizures are the most common indication for EEG. Most of patients performed routine EEG, with a few cases submitted to continuous video-EEG monitoring [42, 58]. A systematic review found that continuous EEG studies reported more abnormalities than routine EEG [59].

Even though EEG abnormalities are frequent, none of available studies showed specific findings in COVID-19 patients. The most commonly described abnormalities are diffuse slow activity (accounting for 60% of findings in these patients) and, less frequently, focal slow activity [56]. One study showed that brain reactivity was reduced or absent more often in COVID-19 patients with poor prognosis [27, 60]. Confusion and seizures seem to be the most frequent predictors of encephalopathy [58].

According to available literature, epileptiform abnormalities and periodic patterns account for 13–20% of EEG findings in COVID-19 patients, more often found in critically ill patients and in those whose presented seizures [42, 56, 59]. Several EEG patterns were reported in status epilepticus (SE) associated to COVID-19, including periodic discharges (lateralized, bilateral, and generalized) and rhythmic discharges, but no single pattern appears to be specific. EEG findings localized to frontal lobe were described in almost half of SE [59].

Just a few patients had focal abnormalities explained by structural focal lesions as ischemic stroke, encephalitis, and unspecified gliosis [56].

One report found severity of EEG findings may be correlated with oxygen saturation at admission and with severity of COVID-19 [59]. It is difficult to relate EEG findings with CSF and neuroimaging findings as just a few patients underwent a complete screening for all modalities. One study was able to obtain records of thoracic CT scan, CSF SARS-CoV-2 PCR, and EEG of a subgroup of 13 patients, and no correlations were found between those variables [58].

There are some limitations to obtain information in this field. Timing of EEG is difficult to recall, as it is usually performed according to onset of neurological complication and not COVID-19 classical symptoms. Information about disease severity and anti-seizure medication and sedatives at time of EEG is not always clear [56].

5.3 Neuroimaging findings

Neuroimaging findings in COVID-19 patients are heterogeneous, varying according to disease severity and neurological concomitant complications [42]. Available cases and reviews suggest more than two-thirds of COVID-19 patients, who undergo brain imaging (CT or MRI), do not show abnormalities presumably associated to infection [61].

Among those who present abnormalities, the most common findings were unspecific diffuse white matter (WM) abnormality (accounting for about 75% of reported findings) and acute or subacute ischemic strokes. WM signal abnormality is usually described as subcortical and periventricular, in association with microhemorrhages. Cerebellar, midline, and deep brain structures involvement is uncommon [61, 62]. Leukoaraiosis is one important finding attributable to aging, and one review suggested its prevalence was higher in COVID-19 patients than expected for age. However, relationship between COVID-19 infection and structural brain lesions is not clear yet. Cortical FLAIR signal abnormality was described in a vast differential diagnosis, including patients with encephalitis, post-ictal state, PRES, and acute ischemia [61].

In a cohort of patients with SE, MRI revealed abnormalities in about 43% of patients, mainly inflammatory lesions, and lesions suggestive of PRES, brain atrophy, cerebral hemorrhage, and brain tumor. Inflammatory lesions did not reveal a specific localization nor a specific cortical involvement in most of cases [55].

6. Conclusions

SARS-CoV-2 seems to have neurotropism and neuroinvasion mechanisms, similar to previous known human coronavirus infections, and neurological complications are frequent [22]. Despite of all new information constantly being published about this issue, robust and complete data are lacking about seizures in patients with COVID-19.

Systemic infection may be a trigger for breakthrough seizures in patients with a history of epilepsy and respiratory infection in particular is a well-known precipitant of acute symptomatic seizures in such individuals [27]. Severe systemic illness, metabolic derangements, emotional stress, the eventual inability to obtain anti-seizure drugs (as patients may avoid hospitals and pharmacies and have more difficulty to get their medications), or gastrointestinal symptoms impeding absorption of oral medications are just examples of the diversity of ways through which COVID-19 may be associated with recurrence of seizures in the epileptic population [25, 27]. As any other infectious disease, COVID-19 can present with significant electrolytic and metabolic imbalance, as hyponatremia or uremic state, both potentially responsible for lowering the seizure threshold in susceptible, non-epileptic, patients. Acute symptomatic seizure can also occur in the context of cerebrovascular disease [27].

Nevertheless, seizure occurrence in COVID-19 is uncommon. Most of the available reviews report an incidence lower than 1% of SARS-CoV-2 infections, even lower than that described in previous human coronaviruses. Higher risk is appointed for patients with poor general condition and severe COVID-19 symptoms [26, 27].

Regardless of etiology, COVID-19 should be considered in the differential diagnosis for patients presenting with seizures during the pandemic, as early consideration may lead to earlier detection and appropriate precautions [27]. Particular attention should rise for patients with altered mental status and the risk of nonconvulsive status epilepticus.

Acknowledgements

We dedicate this work to all victims of COVID-19 and their families, as well as to all health professionals specially those working with COVID-19 patients.

Conflict of interest

The authors declare no conflict of interest.

Author details

Rafael Jesus[1], Carolina Azoia[1], Paulo Coelho[2] and Pedro Guimarães[3*]

1 Neurology Department, Centro Hospitalar de Trás-os-Montes e Alto Douro, Vila Real, Portugal

2 Neurology Department, Oporto CUF Hospital, Oporto, Portugal

3 Neurology Department, Neurophysiology Unit - Centro Hospitalar de Trás-os-Montes e Alto Douro, Vila Real, Portugal

*Address all correspondence to: guimaraes.pedro.s@gmail.com

References

[1] McIntosh K. COVID-19: Epidemiology, virology, and prevention. In: Post TW, editor. UpToDate. Waltham, MA: UpToDate Inc; 2021. Available from: https://www.uptodate.com [Accessed on September 12, 2021]

[2] Zhu N, Zhang D, Wang W, Li X, Yang B, et al. A novel coronavirus from patients with pneumonia in China, 2019. The New England Journal of Medicine. 2020;**382**(8):727-733

[3] Lu R, Zhao X, Li J, Niu P, Yang B, et al. Genomic characterisation and epidemiology of 2019 novel coronavirus: Implications for virus origins and receptor binding. Lancet. 2020;**395**: 565-574

[4] Vilcek S. SARS-CoV-2: Zoonotic origin of pandemic coronavirus. Acta Virologica. 2020;**64**(3):281-287

[5] Ni W, Yang X, Yang D, Bao J, Li R, Xiao Y, et al. Role of angiotensin-converting enzyme 2 (ACE2) in COVID-19. Critical Care. BioMed Central. 2020;**24**(1):422

[6] World Health Organization. Coronavirus disease 2019 (COVID- 19): situation report, 61. World Health Organization; 2020. Available from: https://apps.who.int/iris/handle/10665/331605 [Accessed on September 10, 2021]

[7] Román GC, Spencer PS, Reis J, Buguet A, Faris MEA, Katrak SM, et al. The neurology of COVID-19 revisited: A proposal from the environmental neurology specialty Group of the World Federation of neurology to implement international neurological registries. Journal of the Neurological Sciences. 2020;**414**:116884

[8] Asadi-Pooya AA. Seizures associated with coronavirus infections. Seizure. 2020;**79**:49-52

[9] Bridwell R, Long B, Gottlieb M. Neurologic complications of COVID-19. The American Journal of Emergency Medicine. 2020;**38**(7):1549.e3-1549.e7

[10] Wu Y, Xu X, Chen Z, Duan J, Hashimoto K, Yang L, et al. Nervous system involvement after infection with COVID-19 and other coronaviruses. Brain, Behavior, and Immunity. Academic Press Inc. 2020;**87**:18-22

[11] Ellul M, Benjamin L, Singh B, Lant S, Michael B, Kneen R, et al. Neurological associations of COVID-19. SSRN Electronic Journal. 2020;**19**(9):767-783

[12] Yachou Y, El Idrissi A, Belapasov V, Ait BS. Neuroinvasion, neurotropic, and neuroinflammatory events of SARS-CoV-2: Understanding the neurological manifestations in COVID-19 patients. Neurological Sciences. 2020;**41**(10): 2657-2669

[13] Li W, Moore MJ, Vasilieva N, Sui J, Wong SK, Berne MA, et al. Angiotensin-converting enzyme 2 is a functional receptor for the SARS coronavirus. Nature. 2003;**426**(27):450-454

[14] Verdecchia P, Cavallini C, Spanevello A, Angeli F. The pivotal link between ACE2 deficiency and SARS-CoV-2 infection. European Journal of Internal Medicine. 2020;**76**:14-20

[15] Fotuhi M, Mian A, Meysami S, Raji CA. Neurobiology of COVID-19. Journal of Alzheimer's Disease. 2020;**76**(1):3-19

[16] Angeli F, Zappa M, Reboldi G, Trapasso M, Cavallini C, Spanevello A, et al. The pivotal link between ACE2 deficiency and SARS-CoV-2 infection: One year later. European Journal of Internal Medicine. 2021;**93**:28-34

[17] Cagnazzo F, Arquizan C, Derraz I, Dargazanli C, Lefevre PH, Riquelme C,

et al. Neurological manifestations of patients infected with the SARS-CoV-2: A systematic review of the literature. Journal of Neurology. 2021;**268**(8):2656-2665

[18] Lechien JR, Chiesa-Estomba CM, De Siati DR, Horoi M, Le Bon SD, Rodriguez A, et al. Olfactory and gustatory dysfunctions as a clinical presentation of mild-to-moderate forms of the coronavirus disease (COVID-19): A multicenter European study. European Archives of Oto-Rhino-Laryngology. 2020;**277**(8):2251-2261

[19] Meinhardt J, Radke J, Dittmayer C, Franz J, Thomas C, Mothes R, et al. Olfactory transmucosal SARS-CoV-2 invasion as a port of central nervous system entry in individuals with COVID-19. Nature Neuroscience. 2021;**24**(2):168-175

[20] Brann DH, Tsukahara T, Weinreb C, Lipovsek M, Van Den Berge K, Gong B, et al. Non-neuronal expression of SARS-CoV-2 entry genes in the olfactory system suggests mechanisms underlying COVID-19-associated anosmia. Science Advances. 2020;**6**(31):1-20

[21] Payus AO, Lin CLS, Noh MM, Jeffree MS, Ali RA. SARS-CoV-2 infection of the nervous system: A review of the literature on neurological involvement in novel coronavirus disease-(COVID-19). Bosnian Journal of Basic Medical Sciences. 2020;**20**(3): 283-292

[22] Hu J, Jolkkonen J, Zhao C. Neurotropism of SARS-CoV-2 and its neuropathological alterations: Similarities with other coronaviruses. Neuroscience and Biobehavioral Reviews. 2020;**119**:184-193

[23] Garg RK, Paliwal VK, Gupta A. Encephalopathy in patients with COVID-19: A review. Journal of Medical Virology. 2021;**93**(1):206-222

[24] Mao L, Jin H, Wang M, Hu Y, Chen S, He Q, et al. Neurologic manifestations of hospitalized patients with coronavirus disease 2019 in Wuhan, China. JAMA Neurology. 2020;**77**(6):683-690

[25] Kuroda N. Epilepsy and COVID-19: Updated evidence and narrative review. Epilepsy and Behavior. 2021;**116**:107785

[26] Vohora D, Jain S, Tripathi M, Potschka H. COVID-19 and seizures: Is there a link? Epilepsia. 2020;**61**(9): 1840-1853

[27] Anand P, Al-Faraj A, Sader E, Dashkoff J, Abdennadher M, Murugesan R, et al. Seizure as the presenting symptom of COVID-19: A retrospective case series. Epilepsy & Behavior. 2020;**112**:107335

[28] Fasano A, Cavallieri F, Canali E, Valzania F. First motor seizure as presenting symptom of SARS-CoV-2 infection. Neurological Sciences. 2020;**41**(7):1651-1653

[29] Kurd M, Hashavya S, Benenson S, Gilboa T. Seizures as the main presenting manifestation of acute SARS-CoV-2 infection in children. Seizure - European Journal of Epilepsy. 2021;**92**:89-93

[30] Rana A, Musto AE. The role of inflammation in the development of epilepsy. Journal of Neuroinflammation. 2018;**15**(1):144

[31] Alyu F, Dikmen M. Inflammatory aspects of epileptogenesis: Contribution of molecular inflammatory mechanisms. Acta Neuropsychiatrica. 2017;**29**(1):1-16

[32] Nikbakht F, Mohammadkhanizadeh A, Mohammadi E. How does the COVID-19 cause seizure and epilepsy in patients? The potential mechanisms. Multiple Sclerosis and Related Disorders. 2020;**46**:102535

[33] Bronisz E, Kurkowska-Jastrzębska I. Matrix metalloproteinase 9 in epilepsy: The role of Neuroinflammation in seizure development. Mediators of Inflammation. 2016;**2016**:7369020

[34] Coperchini F, Chiovato L, Croce L, Magri F, Rotondi M. The cytokine storm in COVID-19: An overview of the involvement of the chemokine/chemokine-receptor system. Cytokine & Growth Factor Reviews. 2020;**53**:25-32

[35] Castelli V, Cimini A, Ferri C. Cytokine storm in COVID-19: "When you come out of the storm, you Won't Be the same person who walked in." Frontiers in Immunology. 2020;**11**:2132

[36] Sayer JA, Mabillard H. Electrolyte disturbances in SARS-CoV-2 infection. F1000Research. 2020;**9**:587

[37] Lippi G, South AM, Henry BM. Electrolyte imbalances in patients with severe coronavirus disease 2019 (COVID-19). Annals of Clinical Biochemistry. 2020;**57**(3):262-265

[38] Nardone R, Brigo F, Trinka E. Acute symptomatic seizures caused by electrolyte disturbances. Journal of Clinical Neurology. 2016;**12**(1):21

[39] Marazuela M, Giustina A, Puig-Domingo M. Endocrine and metabolic aspects of the COVID-19 pandemic. Reviews in Endocrine & Metabolic Disorders. 2020;**21**(4):1

[40] Beleza P. Acute symptomatic seizures: A clinically oriented review. The Neurologist. 2012;**18**(3):109-119

[41] Parauda SC, Gao V, Gewirtz AN, Parikh NS, Merkler AE, Lantos J, et al. Posterior reversible encephalopathy syndrome in patients with COVID-19. Journal of the Neurological Sciences. 2020;**416**:117019

[42] Hwang ST, Ballout AA, Mirza U, Sonti AN, Husain A, Kirsch C, et al. Acute seizures occurring in association with SARS-CoV-2. Frontiers in Neurology. 2020;**11**:576329

[43] Connors JM, Levy JH. COVID-19 and its implications for thrombosis and anticoagulation. Blood. 2020;**135**(23):2033-2040

[44] Tang N, Li D, Wang X, Sun Z. Abnormal coagulation parameters are associated with poor prognosis in patients with novel coronavirus pneumonia. Journal of Thrombosis and Haemostasis. 2020;**18**(4):844-847

[45] Vogrig A, Gigli GL, Bnà C, Morassi M. Stroke in patients with COVID-19: Clinical and neuroimaging characteristics. Neuroscience Letters. 2021;**743**:135564

[46] Reddy DS, Bhimani A, Kuruba R, Park MJ, Sohrabji F. Prospects of modeling poststroke epileptogenesis. Journal of Neuroscience Research. 2017;**95**(4):1000-1016

[47] Guo CY, Sun L, Chen XP, Zhang DS. Oxidative stress, mitochondrial damage and neurodegenerative diseases. Neural Regeneration Research. 2013;**8**(21):2003

[48] Silva B, Jorge A, Luzeiro I. Neurologic manifestations in sars-cov-2 infected patients. Sinapse. 2020;**20**(2): 9-16

[49] Sutter R, Rüegg S, Tschudin-Sutter S. Seizures as adverse events of antibiotic drugs: A systematic review. Neurology. 2015;**85**(15):1332-1341

[50] Lu L, Xiong W, Liu D, Liu J, Yang D, Li N, et al. New onset acute symptomatic seizure and risk factors in coronavirus disease 2019: A retrospective multicenter study. Epilepsia. 2020;**61**(6):e49-e53

[51] Hung E, Chim S, Chan P, Tong Y, Ng E, Chiu R, et al. Detection of SARS coronavirus RNA in the cerebrospinal

fluid of a patient with severe acute respiratory syndrome. Clinical Chemistry. 2003;**49**:2108-2109

[52] Asadi-Pooya AA, Simani L, Shahisavandi M, Barzegar Z. COVID-19, de novo seizures, and epilepsy: A systematic review. Neurological Sciences. 2021;**42**(2):415-431

[53] Emami A, Fadakar N, Akbari A, Lotfi M, Farazdaghi M, Javanmardi F, et al. Seizure in patients with COVID-19. Neurological Sciences. 2020;**41**(11): 3057-3061

[54] Kadono Y, Nakamura Y, Ogawa Y, Yamamoto S, Kajikawa R, Nakajima Y, et al. A case of COVID-19 infection presenting with a seizure following severe brain edema. Seizure. 2020;**80**: 53-55

[55] Dono F, Nucera B, Lanzone J, Evangelista G, Rinaldi F, Speranza R, et al. Status epilepticus and COVID-19: A systematic review. Epilepsy & Behavior. 2021;**118**:107887

[56] Roberto KT, Espiritu AI, Fernandez MLL, Gutierrez JC. Electroencephalographic findings in COVID-19 patients: A systematic review. Seizure. 2020;**82**:17-22

[57] Carroll E, Melmed KR, Frontera J, Placantonakis DG, Galetta S, Balcer L, et al. Cerebrospinal fluid findings in patients with seizure in the setting of COVID-19: A review of the literature. Seizure. 2021;**89**:99-106

[58] Besnard S, Nardin C, Lyon E, Debroucker T, Arjmand R, Moretti R, et al. Electroencephalographic Abnormalites in SARS-CoV-2 patients. Frontiers in Neurology. 2020;**11**:582794

[59] Antony AR, Haneef Z. Systematic review of EEG findings in 617 patients diagnosed with COVID-19. Seizure. 2020;**83**:234-241

[60] Pati S, Toth E, Chaitanya G. Quantitative EEG markers to prognosticate critically ill patients with COVID-19: A retrospective cohort study. Clinical Neurophysiology. 2020;**131**(8):1824

[61] Egbert AR, Cankurtaran S, Karpiak S. Brain abnormalities in COVID-19 acute/subacute phase: A rapid systematic review. Brain, Behavior, and Immunity. 2020;**89**: 543-554

[62] Gulko E, Oleksk ML, Gomes W, Ali S, Mehta H, Overby P, et al. MRI brain findings in 126 patients with COVID-19: Initial observations from a descriptive literature review. AJNR. American Journal of Neuroradiology. 2020;**41**(12):2199-2203

Section 2

Molecular and Cellular Neurochemistry

Chapter 4

Peripheral Biomarkers in Multiple Sclerosis Patients Treated with Interferon-Beta

Andreia Monteiro, Ana Mafalda Fonseca and Artur Paiva

Abstract

Multiple sclerosis is a relapsing and eventually progressive disorder of the central nervous system that continues to challenge researchers who try to understand the pathogenesis of the disease and prevent its progression. Interferon-beta is the most widely prescribed treatment for MS. Peripheral blood seems to mirror the immunological disturbances that underlie MS, which could represent the migration patterns between periphery and other tissues according to the clinical phase of the disease. Based on this assumption, several studies point to significant alterations in peripheral blood homeostasis of different subpopulations of T cells, like γδ T cells or Th1, Th2 and Th17 functional subsets; of B cells subpopulations; and of innate cells like monocytes and dendritic cells. The main goal of this chapter is to make an in-depth review of the major findings described in the literature that correlate specific alterations on different leukocytes subpopulations with disease status, and which therefore have the potential to constitute a peripheral biomarker of disease progression.

Keywords: biomarkers, T cells, B cells, dendritic cells, monocytes

1. Introduction

Around 2.8 million people are diagnosed with multiple sclerosis (MS) worldwide. MS is an autoimmune demyelinating disease of the central nervous system (CNS) of unknown etiology. Hallmarks of MS include focal inflammatory infiltrates, demyelinating plaques, reactive gliosis, and axonal damage [1, 2].

The mechanism of MS pathology involves complex interactions between systems and cell types including neurons, glia, and immune cells, accompanied by permeability of the blood–brain barrier (BBB). Autoreactive T cells activated outside the CNS cross the BBB and are reactivated by local antigen-presenting cells. Secretion of proinflammatory cytokines stimulates microglial cells and astrocytes, recruits additional inflammatory cells, and induces antibody production by plasma cells [3].

Recombinant interferon-β (IFN-β) remains the most widely prescribed treatment for relapsing–remitting MS (RRMS) and a valid approach because of its good benefit/risk profile. Despite widespread use of IFN-β, its therapeutic mechanism is still partially understood. The efficacy of IFN-β treatment has been shown by a decreased annual relapse rate, disability progression and inflammatory brain lesions resulting in the approval of different IFN-β preparations [4].

IFN-β is a highly pleiotropic cytokine which antagonizes the proinflammatory milieu by inhibiting expression of proinflammatory molecules, while increasing production of anti-inflammatory factors. It inhibits leukocyte trafficking, regulates the adhesion molecule expression and inhibits matrix metalloproteinase activity. The mechanism of action of IFN-β is complex and multifactorial but has been shown to reduce the biological activity of RRMS in several clinical class I trials [5].

The identification of peripheral markers that could reflect the clinical course of MS and the efficacy of treatment is a stimulating field of research and debate. An ideal biomarker is characterized by high sensitivity and specificity as well as a simple, cost effective, reproducible, and non-invasive detection method [6]. For instance, there are reports focusing molecules and autoantibodies as potential biomarkers in the MS disease course. Our focus in this chapter is on circulating leucocytes that can be considered during the follow of RRMS patients in remission *versus* relapse phase.

2. Multiple sclerosis

MS is an autoimmune disease of the brain and the spinal cord characterized by chronic inflammation, demyelination, gliosis and neuronal loss. The demyelination consists of the damage of the myelin sheath surrounding nerves, consequently affects the function of the nerves. The pathological hallmark of chronic MS is the demyelinated plaque or lesions, which consists of a well-demarcated hypocellular area characterized by the loss of myelin sheaths or oligodendrocytes, relative preservation of axons, and the formation of astrocytic scars [1].

The etiology of MS remains elusive, with a complex multifactorial system implicated, in which environmental factors are hypothesized as interacting with genetically susceptible individuals. MS causes a heterogeneous array of symptoms and signs because of the differential involvement of motor, sensory, visual and autonomic systems with serious physical disability in young adults, especially women [2, 4, 7].

The CNS is frequently described as an immune-privileged site, evidence supports the notion that the CNS receives limited immune surveillance by peripheral lymphocytes under physiological conditions. New findings provide a mechanism by which large particles and immune cells can drain from the brain and interface directly with the peripheral immune system [8, 9].

MS is triggered in the periphery or in the CNS. The CNS-extrinsic (peripheral) model is the most widely accepted and is consistent with the method used to induce experimental autoimmune encephalomyelitis (EAE), the animal model for neuroinflammation. The autoreactive T cells from MS patients may become activated in the periphery as a result of a molecular mimicry, gain access to the CNS, and T cells generated against non-self-epitopes (viral or microbial antigens) cross-react with self-myelin epitopes of similar sequence [10–12].

85% of patients present a RR form of MS, characterized by discrete episodes of neurological dysfunction (relapses) separated by clinical stable periods with lack of disease progression (remissions). More than 30% remain in the RRMS form of the disease into old age [7, 11–13].

Relapse is the clinical result of an acute inflammatory focal lesion and is typically discernible using magnetic resonance imaging. Relapse is defined as newly appearing neurological symptoms in the absence of fever or infections that last for more than 24 hours and are separated from the previous event by at least one month. The frequency of relapses can vary widely among patients as well as during different periods during an individual patient's disease. The relapse tends to be present for a limited time – days or weeks – and can lead to full recovery or can leave sequelae.

At present time, no clinical features or biomarkers that are predictive of relapse rates have been identified. The signs and symptoms that occur during relapses are also diverse and unpredictable [3, 8, 11].

Immunological characteristics of MS lesions have been reflected in circulating immune cells of MS patients. Peripheral blood provides a 'window' into the immunopathogenesis of MS. The immunological disturbances that underlie MS can be observed not only in the CNS, but also through examination of peripheral immune cells [14].

3. Therapeutic management

IFN-β and glatiramer acetate have been used as first-line disease-modifying therapy for RRMS. More than two decades have passed since IFN-β was found to be effective in the management of MS. IFN-β treatment efficacy has been shown by a decrease in the annual relapse rate, in disability progression and in inflammatory brain lesions, resulting in the approval of different IFN-β preparations [15–17]·

IFNs are naturally occurring cytokines, secreted by various cells such as fibroblasts, NK cells, leukocytes, and epithelial cells in response to pathogens such as bacteria, viruses, parasites, and tumor cells, as well as other foreign substances. They have a wide range in anti-inflammatory processes, regulation of cell growth and modulation of immune responses [18, 19].

IFN-β binds to the interferon receptor, activates the Janus kinase/signal transducer and the activator of transcription (STAT) pathway to phosphorylate STAT1 and STAT2. The activation of interferon-stimulated genes leads to the production of antiviral, antiproliferative, and antitumour products. The effectiveness of IFN-β in the treatment of MS may rely on both anti-viral and immunomodulatory aspects [20, 21].

IFN-β was the first immunomodulatory therapy approved by the U.S. Food and Drug Administration and is the most widely prescribed treatment for MS; it is generally well tolerated and overall reduces the relapse rate by 30% in patients with RRMS [4].

Several IFN-β preparations have been approved with differing structures (glycosylated IFN-β-1a vs. non-glycosylated IFN-β-1b), formulation (lyophilized vs. liquid), used excipients (e.g., containing serum albumin or not), modification (pegylation), dosage (protein load and bioactivity), route of administration (subcutaneous vs. intramuscular), or frequency of injection (ranging from bi-weekly to every other day). IFN-β shows high tissue distribution; however, it is not supposed to cross the BBB and exerts its immunomodulatory mechanism in the peripheral compartment. IFN-β is cleared via renal and hepatic pathways, in which catabolism seems to be important rather than simple excretion [15]·

The therapeutic benefit of IFN-β in MS has been proven in several large clinical trials, with the effect of IFN-β therapy being more studied on T and B cells [22]. In spite of this, it is known that the biological functions of IFN-β act in both innate and adaptive immune responses and may influence phenotype and functions of all MS-relevant immune cells [23].

4. Peripheral blood leukocytes as potential biomarkers of disease activity

A biomarker is defined as a characteristic that can be objectively measured and evaluated and serves as an indicator of normal biological processes, pathological processes or pharmacological reactions to therapy. An ideal biomarker is characterized by high sensitivity and specificity as well as a simple, cost effective, reproducible, and non-invasive detection method [6].

In this section we synthesize and integrate the most relevant data regarding the characteristics of the selected immune cells that could be considered as IFN-β treatment-related biomarkers. The main goal of this work is an attempt to help researchers to perform a good assessment of immune cells in future studies. The presented data is a result of a compilation of several studies and findings.

4.1 Antigen-presenting cells

Antigen presenting cells (APCs) are considered key players in the immune surveillance of CNS and, at the same time, they are critically involved in the pathogenesis of CNS autoimmune diseases. They are a morphologically and functionally diverse group of cells that links the innate and adaptive immune responses. These cells are specialized in the presentation of antigens to lymphocytes, particularly T cells. Included among such cells are dendritic cells (DCs), monocytes and macrophages (derived from monocytes that migrated from the blood stream to tissues). B lymphocytes that specifically capture antigens via their clonally expressed membrane immunoglobulin can also function efficiently as APCs to T cells [24].

4.1.1 Dendritic cells

In humans, DCs comprise two major subsets: plasmacytoid DCs (pDCs) and myeloid (mDCs). Through nucleic acid-sensing, pDCs activate toll-like receptors (TLR), such as TLR7 and TLR9, rapidly producing type I IFN. mDCs are dedicated APCs that have a characteristic dendritic morphology, express high levels of MHC class II molecules and recognize pathogen-derived lipids, proteins and nucleic-acids by TLR2, TLR4 and TLR3 respectively [25].

The DCs subsets may be helpful as biomarker between remission and relapse of RRMS patients treated with IFN-β. The circulating mDCs subset reduces in remission and increase in relapse RRMS patients. On the other hand, the pDCs frequency are maintain across the different phases of disease. Usually, these subsets present a low frequency in systemic circulation, so the mDCs/pDCs ratio is a good representative of the alteration observed in the DCs subsets. The mDCs/pDCs decreases in remission RRMS patients and is re-established in relapse RRMS patients, constituting a potential peripheral biomarker [26, 27].

The involvement of DCs in MS arises from studies that demonstrate the abundant presence of these cells in the inflamed CNS lesions and in the CSF of MS patients [23].

One of the immunomodulatory effects of IFN-β in the EAE model is the reduction in antigen presentation, particularly myelin-specific antigens, leading to reduced T-cell responses [25, 28]. In contrast with these effects, in remission phase it was observed that the DCs subsets increase the expression of HLA-DR and decrease in the relapse phase. The variation in HLA-DR expression is more evident in the mDCs subset. The same subset reduce the mRNA gene expression of CX3CR1; fractalkine is known to be upregulated and released in response to pro-inflammatory stimuli and induces adhesion, chemoattraction, and activation of leukocytes [27].

The activation status of the mDCs subset could discriminate between RRMS phases. This subset shown a highest activated status in remission than in relapse phase, through the increased HLA-DR expression and a reduced migratory capability, since reduce the mRNA gene expression of CX3CR1.

4.1.2 Monocytes

Monocytes represent a heterogeneous population of primary immune effector cells with distinct phenotypical and functional characteristics; their differential roles in steady-state immune surveillance and the pathogenesis of human CNS disease are poorly understood [20].

The differential expression of CD14 (part of the receptor for lipopolysaccharide) and CD16 (also known as FcγRIII) allows monocytes to be segregated into three subsets. The major subset designated "classical" monocytes ($CD14^{++}CD16^{-}$, cMo), corresponds to 80–90% of circulating monocytes. CD16 expressing monocytes are divided into a named "intermediate" monocyte ($CD14^{++}CD16^{+}$, iMo) and a subset classified as "non-classical" monocytes ($CD14^{+}CD16^{++}$, ncMo); each of these subsets corresponds to 5–10% of circulating monocytes [21, 29].

Patients with MS display high levels of monocyte-secreted inflammatory molecules in serum compared to healthy individuals, demonstrating a role for peripheral monocytes in the progression of the disease. Increased levels of serum tumor necrosis factor (TNF) α and β have been reported in MS relapse. Monocytes and microglia are known to act as major effectors in the demyelinating process through direct interaction and the production of proinflammatory cytokines and mediators (e.g., IL-1b, nitric oxide). $CD16^{+}$ monocytes may contribute to the breakdown of the BBB by facilitating T cell trafficking into the CNS [20, 24, 30].

Research performed on monocyte pool in RRMS patients is scarce and ambiguous. A recent work achieved a significant decrease of the ncMo subset in both phases of RRMS patients, although in a higher extension in remission patients [27].

The frequency of monocytes subsets does not allow us to identify different phases of RRMS, but the HLA-DR expression could constitute a potential important biomarker between remission and relapse phases. A significant increase in HLA-DR expression in all monocyte subsets in the remission group when compared with healthy and relapse groups, has been described [27]. IFN-β enhances HLA-DR expression in circulating monocytes, but inside the CNS, one prominent model is based on the observation that IFN-β inhibits the IFNγ upregulation of MHC class II molecules on cell surface of macrophages and glial cells and therefore diminishes antigen presentation [28]. In the periphery, Kantor et al. report that the increase of MHC Class II expression in monocytes induced by IFN-β may contribute to the positive immunomodulatory effect in MS [31]. These findings were reinforced by the observation that when IFN-β-stimulated monocytes were used to stimulate autologous T cells, there was an increased secretion of anti-inflammatory cytokine IL-13 [32].

4.2 T cells

4.2.1 $CD4^{+}$ and $CD8^{+}$ T cells

T cells are central regulators of the adaptive immune response, they help B lymphocytes to produce antibodies and secrete cytokines that provide efficient protection against pathogens. Distinct T helper (Th) cell subsets, producing one or more lineage-defining cytokines and expressing master transcription factors and homing receptors. Th subsets are differentiated from naive $CD4^{+}$ T cells in response to a specific class of pathogenic microorganisms and to the cytokine milieu. This occurs in peripheral lymph nodes by mature DCs that present pathogen-derived peptides associated to MHC class II. With the involvement of their costimulatory molecules, DCs promote T cell proliferation and produce polarizing cytokines. In turn T cell was differentiated in distinct Th cell subsets, such as Th1, Th2, Th17, regulatory T (T reg) and T follicular helper (Tfh) [33].

The $CD4^+$ T cells have been the most studied in the pathogenesis of MS, although $CD8^+$ T cells are the dominant lymphocyte population in all stages of disease and lesions of MS patients. Naive $CD8^+$ T cells follow a similar differentiation programme of $CD4^+$ T cells [34, 35].

Th1 cells are described as being the pathogenic subset of T cells, whereas Th2 cells are reported to exert inhibitory effects [5]. Previous studies have pointed to a reduction in pro-inflammatory capability promoted by IFN-β therapy, consisting of a reduction of the expression of Th1-induced cytokines while enhancing Th2 responses [18]. Concerning the T cytotoxic (Tc) subsets, it has been reported the same behavior, in remission a downregulation of pro-inflammatory Tc1 responses and up-regulation of anti-inflammatory Tc2 with a beneficial effect on disease activity [36]. This dichotomy Th1, Th2 subsets and Tc1, Tc2 subsets could contribute to discriminate between remission and relapse phases.

The identification of Th17 cells helped to resolve some in adequacies of the original Th1/Th2 concept that had dominated T cell immunology research filed for almost 20 years. For a long time, it was thought that the IL-12/IFNγ pathway and Th1 cells were central to the development of autoimmune disease [37].

Both Th1 and Th17 cells have been implicated in the initiation and progression of disease in RRMS and its experimental model EAE [19]. The link between Th17 cells, IL-17 and MS relapses comes from the observation that in humans, Th17 cells are able to cross the BBB in MS lesions, enhancing neuroinflammation. In vitro studies have revealed that IL-17 blocks the differentiation and reduces the survival of oligodendrocyte lineage cells. In EAE model, it has been suggested that Th17 cells interact directly with neurons, forming antigen-independent, immune, synapse-like contacts [7, 38].

It is assumed that the inhibition of Th17 cells in RRMS patients attenuates the disease, however conflicting data have been published. Axtell et al. reported that IFN-β treatment effectively blocked disease symptoms in mice with EAE induced with Th1 cells. Otherwise, in EAE induced with Th17 cells the IFN-β treatment worsened disease [19].

In RRMS patients, it is not clear whether a more specific blockade of the Th17 pathway has beneficial effects in MS patients. Treatment with an antibody directed against IL-12p40 and therefore neutralizing both IL-12 and IL-23 did not result in a significant reduction of disease activity [39].

A meta-analysis pointed out several limitations across studies that assess the levels of peripheral Th17 cells and serum Th17-related cytokines. Like the severities of the disease and clinical subtypes in MS patients; the disease duration from relapse; and that the MS treatments were not consistent; and it was postulated that most studies selected MS patients with high disease activity. There were differences in experimental methods between studies and a lack of detailed standardized methods to identify the Th17 cells and Th17-related cytokines [40].

A recent in vivo study observed an increased frequency of circulating Th17 and Tc17 cells, accompanied by increased serum levels of IL-17 in remission RRMS patients treated with IFN-β [41]. This contradiction underlines the need to clarify the role of the IL-17-producing T cells in RRMS patients.

It has been demonstrated that a significant proportion of Th17 cells convert into IFN-γ-producing T cells and have chemokine receptors from both Th17 and Th1 subtypes, referred as Th17.1 cells. The enhanced potential of Th17.1 cells to infiltrate the CNS was supported by their predominance in CSF of early MS patients and their preferential transmigration across human brain endothelial layers [42, 43]. In remission RRMS patients, it was observed that Th17 and Tc17 cells exhibited a higher degree of Th1 plasticity since there were higher frequencies of those cells simultaneously producing intracellular IL-17 and IL-2 or IFNγ or TNFα [41].

Another subset of T cells, the Tregs, are characterized by high expression of CD25 and the transcription factor *Foxp3*, which is critical for their development, lineage commitment, and regulatory functions. Tregs are a very heterogeneous population with suppressive functions that maintain tolerance to harmless food/self-antigens and prevent autoimmune disease. Numerous studies have identified Tregs as important immunoregulators in many inflammatory and autoimmune disease conditions including asthma, MS, and type-I diabetes [37, 44].

In MS patients, both reduced or normal frequency of Tregs was observed. Libera et al. described a significant decrease in Treg cells in remission RRMS patients [45]. Haas et al. state that the frequency of Treg cells was normal in MS patients but with a lower suppressive function on autoreactive T cells [46]. Venken et al. described that RRMS patients treated with IFN-β showed restored naive Treg numbers as compared with age- and disease-duration-matched untreated patients [47].

Recently identified, the Tfh subset expresses the chemokine receptor CXCR5 as well as CD279 [48], is specialized in helping B cells to produce antibodies in the face of antigenic challenge and plays a crucial role in orchestrating the humoral arm of adaptive immune responses. Tfh cells have the unique ability to migrate into follicles in secondary lymphoid organs where they colocalize with B cells to deliver contact-dependent and soluble signals that support survival and differentiation of the latter cells. There is no complete and thorough understanding of how naïve Th cells differentiate into mature Tfh [49, 50].

Tfh cell levels are elevated in the blood of MS patients and this population is positively correlated with the progression of disability. One potential mechanism through which Tfh cells can contribute to disease is promoting the inflammatory B-cell activities, suggesting that Tfh cells cooperate with Th17 cells to induce inflammatory B cell responses in the CNS and increase disease severity [49].

The increased frequencies of Th1 cells, activated Tfh- and B-cells parallel findings from pathology studies, along with the correlation between activated Tfh- and B-cells, suggest a pathogenic role of systemic inflammation in progressive MS [51].

A similar frequency of Tfh cells between RRMS patients and healthy subjects was reported. However, this subset tend to exhibit a more proinflammatory activity, since higher frequencies of TNF-α^{+} Tfh cells have been observed [41]. It is well known that Tfh cells play an important role in T/B interactions in germinal centres (GC) and one potential mechanism through which Tfh cells can contribute to MS is in promoting inflammatory B-cell activities [49]. The Tfh subset and others follicular like T cells subsets, like Treg/follicular cells, are promising targets in the study of T cells in pathophysiology of MS.

4.2.2 γδ T cells

γδ T cells develop in the thymus together with αβ T cells but rearrange a different TCR, consisting of a TCR-γ and TCR-δ chain. One of the most striking characteristics of γδ T cells is their inherent ability to secrete pro-inflammatory cytokines very rapidly, which influences adaptive immunity, they carry out immediate effector functions as well as mounting a memory response upon microbial reinfection. This fast response can be explained by γδ T cells exiting the thymus already with the functional competence to produce cytokines with no need of APCs cells [52, 53].

In MS, their potential importance is increased by the finding that γδ T cells accumulate in demyelinating CNS MS plaques; these cells show evidence of oligoclonal expansion indicating a local response to currently unknown antigens. γδ T cells have been shown to be present in both MS lesions and in CSF, and sequencing studies have shown that the major γδ T subsets present in the lesion differ from those in the CSF, suggesting specific functions for these cells in lesion development.

In more chronic lesions, γδ T cells may become the most prevalent type of T cell in the lesion. γδ T cells isolated from the CNS can be expanded but only in patients with relapse disease, not chronic MS patients, suggesting that these cells may have differential roles during various phases of the disease [54, 55].

The frequency, the migratory pattern, the activation status of γδ T cells in RRMS patients are unclear. Between remission and relapse RRMS patients, the γδ terminally differentiated effector memory T cells (T_{EMRA}) and the $CCR5^{+}$ γδ T_{EMRA} decrease in relapse when compared with remission RRMS patients [56], constituting a good biomarker between phases of the disease. Probably as a result of the migratory pattern describe for this phase of MS, preferentially toward RANTES and MIP-1α, whose expression is increased during relapses [57, 58].

The decrease of Eomesodermin and granzyme B mRNA expression in $CD27^{-}$ γδ T cells suggests a reduction in the cytotoxic potential of the circulating pool of γδ T cells, particularly in relapsing RRMS patients [56].

4.3 B lymphocytes

The most consistent immunodiagnostic feature and hallmark immunologic finding in MS patients is the presence of oligoclonal bands (OCB) in the CSF and their absence in peripheral circulation. Consequently, the pathogenic function of B cells in MS has been traditionally associated with antibody production. However, B cells have three putative biological roles: production of proinflammatory or regulatory cytokines, function as APCs and antibody production [59].

In MS, the memory B cells, plasmablasts and plasma cells preferentially cross the BBB and migrate into the CNS, where they dominate the B cell pool and exert different effector functions. B cells seem to be abnormally polarized toward a more proinflammatory phenotype [60].

More recent, somatic hypermutation studies have demonstrated that identical B cell clones can be shared between the CNS and the periphery in individual patients. These studies provide evidence of bidirectional trafficking of distinct B cell clones (both into and out of the CNS). The patterns suggest that B cells can travel back and forth across the BBB and commonly re-enter GC (in the meninges or cervical lymph nodes) to undergo further somatic hypermutations. These findings change our view of lymphocytic surveillance of CNS tissue and underline that B-cell trafficking is an important topic for future research and therapy strategies [60–62]. This news about recirculation of B cells through the BBB alters the perception of the role of B cells in MS.

B cells are released in the peripheral blood, recirculate between the secondary lymphoid tissues, and dying after a few days. According to phenotypic profile of B cell subsets, which also reflects their functional abilities and behavior, four major maturation-associated subsets can be identified in the human peripheral blood: immature/transitional, naive, memory and plasmablast [63].

In remission RRMS patients submitted to IFN-β, the percentage of immature/transitional B cells increases. This increase can be seen as an attempt to increase anti-inflammatory cytokines. Meanwhile, a decrease in the proportion of circulating class-switched memory B cells was reported [64, 65].

The relapsing RRMS patients exhibited distinct changes in B cell subsets homeostasis, resulting in a decrease in the total population of B cells, including a decrease of the immature/transitional and naïve B cell subsets when compared with remission RRMS patients. On the other hand, the plasmablast B cell subset presented an increase in relapse RRMS patients. The ratio between immature/transitional B cells and plasmablasts can thus be considered as a potential biomarker between phases of RRMS patients. The remission RRMS patients and the healthy subjects presented a similar ratio, and the relapse RRMS patients present a decreased ratio [66].

According to the new and recent data about the recirculation of B cells in RRMS, it seems that the increase of plasmablasts in circulation of relapsing episodes may be due to a migration of these cells from cervical lymph nodes and/or from B cell aggregates described in the meninges of MS patients to the blood marrow in an attempt to promote the immune response [67].

5. Effects of IFN-β in circulating cells

An ever-expanding body of literature, sometimes difficult to integrate, defines the intricate pathways by which IFN-β mediates its broad effects. To resume the effects of IFN-β in circulating immune cells a table listing the relevant studies and findings was performed (**Table 1**).

	Effects of IFN-β
Antigen presenting cells	• reduces mDCs frequency, pDCs frequency remains unchanged, mDCs/pDCs ratio decreases [25, 27, 65]; • activated pDCs decreased TLR9 consequently decreases Th1 cell differentiation, reduced pro-inflammatory IL-6, TNF-α, IFNγ secretion, expression of CCR7 and increased IL-10 secretion [20, 25–27, 66] • activated status mDCs trough the expression of HLA-DR and mRNA gene expression of CX3CR1 reducing their migration pattern [27] • pDCs showed reduced expression of the maturation markers CD83 and CD86 molecules and lower secretion of proinflammatory cytokines, including IFN-α, and a decreased ability to stimulate allogeneic T cells in response to maturation stimuli [24, 65]; • enhances HLA-DR expression in circulating monocytes [27, 28]
T cells	• reduces T-cell activation, downregulating MHC class II and costimulatory molecules, prevents the interaction of B7/CD28 and CD40/CD40L decreases the activation of myelin-reactive T cells [4, 5, 25]; • inhibits proinflammatory IFNγ, TNFα and IL-17, increasing the production of IL-10 [5, 68]; • increases levels of Th1 cytokines during RRMS relapse, whereas Th2 cytokines increases during remission in RRMS patients [5, 25, 40]; • prevents T-cell adhesion and extravasation across the BBB [4, 5]; • induces Treg cells [4, 5, 22]; • Mediates the chemokine receptor CCR7, channel autoreactive T cells into secondary lymphoid tissue rather than to CNS [5]; • the $CCR5^{+}\gamma\delta$ T_{EMRA} cells decreases with a reduction in the cytotoxic potential in relapse when compared to remission [56]
B cells	• induces expression of the B-cell survival factor B-cell-activating factor, with a shift toward less mature circulating B cells [65]; • reduces of memory B cell frequency exerted by the induction of a FAS-R-mediated caspase 3-dependent apoptosis [16]; • downregulates costimulatory molecules, CD40 and CD80 becoming less efficient APCs and less able to induce T-cell proliferation [23]; • inhibits proinflammatory cytokines, IL-1β and IL-23, anti-inflammatory IL-10 is upregulated in B cells [24, 64]; • the ratio between immature/transitional B cells and plasmablasts decreases in relapse when compared to remission RRMS [66]

Table 1.
Main effects of IFN-β in circulating immune cells in MS.

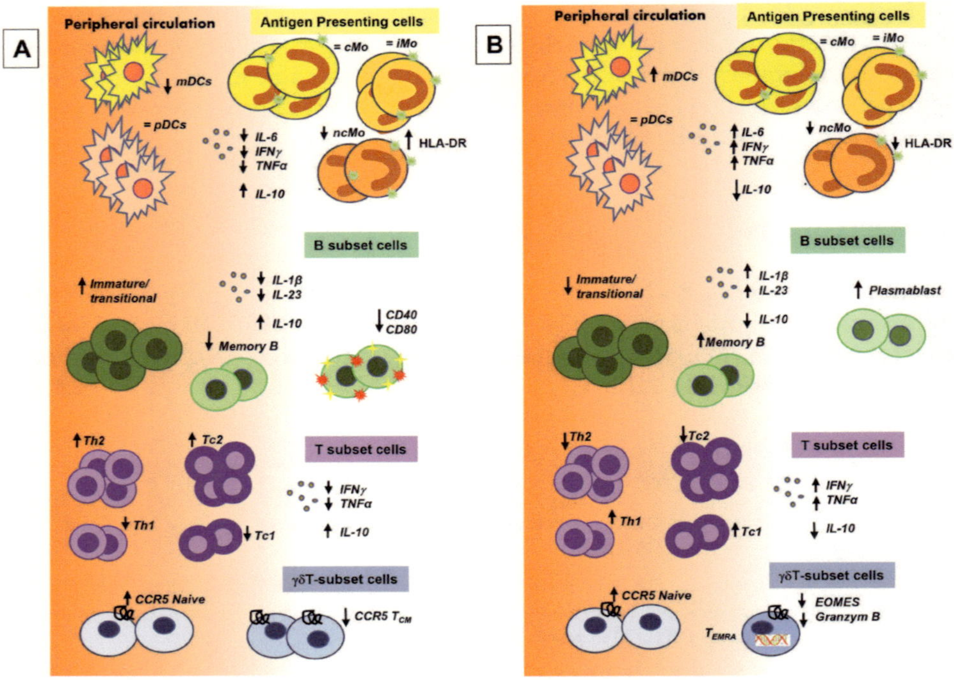

Figure 1.
Main effects of IFN-β in RRMS patients (a) remission phase and (B) relapse phase. mDC – Myeloid dendtitic, pDC – Plasmacytoid dendtitic cell, cMO – Classical monocytes, iMo – Intermediate monocytes, ncMo – Non-classical monocytes.

A major role for IFN-β is the induction of a priming state through which production and regulation of mediators, including cytokines, are affected by synergistic or antagonistic interactions. In the treatment of MS, the most important IFN-β mechanisms of action appear to be mediated mainly by the increased expression and concentration of anti-inflammatory agents, in turn, down-regulating the inflammatory state observed in the patients both in the periphery and in the brain tissue (**Figure 1**) [23].

6. Methodology

The work from our group started with the selection of the RRMS patients and collected blood from each one after assigned an informed consent. By flow cytometry performed direct immunofluorescence membrane and intracytoplasmic staining protocols to identify and characterize the circulating subsets. To functional assessment of the cells was measured intracellular cytokines at single cell level, after in vitro stimulation. To evaluation of gene expression, RNA isolation and quantitative real-time reverse transcriptase-polymerase chain reaction was performed.

In our group publications, one can be find the flow strategy with the description of the antibodies used and the mRNA gene expression studies performed in APCs [27], in T cell subsets [41], in γδ T cells [56] and in B cell subsets [66].

The literature search was performed using the PubMed electronic bibliographic database. The search was restricted to English and publications between 2010 and 2021. The keywords used were: multiple sclerosis, IFN-β, antigen presenting cells, T cells and B cells alone or in conjugation. The bibliographies of retrieved articles and previous review articles were hand searched to obtain additional articles.

DOI: http://dx.doi.org/10.5772/intechopen.99006

7. Conclusion

In demyelinating diseases, mainly in relapse phase of RRMS, the BBB suffer a profound disturbance, so as the exchanges and ultimately the CNS itself. Despite CNS suffered an immune response, immune abnormalities could be found in the peripheral immune compartment.

The periphery assumes an extremely important role in the study of MS. In remission phase is establish an equilibrium between CNS and systemic circulation. In this chapter we have attempted to contribute to highlight the more relevant data regarding circulating cell subsets that could potentially be considered as peripheral biomarkers in RRMS patients treated with IFN-β.

Some circulating immune cells assume differences between the remission and relapse phases of RRMS. These differences may be used as disease activity biomarkers to measure inflammatory and/or neurodegenerative components of disease and helpful to discriminate between phases of RRMS.

Technological advances of flow cytometry have greatly increased the strength of analysis achievable at the single-cell level. These developments can be applied to understand more clearly the immunopathology of MS and the identification of consistent, safe and reproducible biomarkers in the periphery.

Funding

This work was financed by the Foundation for Science and Technology (FCT), through funds from the State Budget, and by the European Regional Development Fund (ERDF), under the Portugal 2020 Program, through the Regional Operational Program of the Center (Centro2020), through the Project with the reference UIDB/00709/2020.

Author details

Andreia Monteiro[1,2*], Ana Mafalda Fonseca[1] and Artur Paiva[3,4,5]

1 CICS-UBI—Health Sciences Research Centre, University of Beira Interior, Covilhã, Portugal

2 Clinical Pathology Service, Centro Hospitalar Universitário da Cova da Beira Covilhã, Portugal

3 Cytometry Operational Management Unit, Clinical Pathology Service, Centro Hospitalar e Universitário de Coimbra, Coimbra, Portugal

4 Coimbra Institute for Clinical and Biomedical Research (iCBR), Medicine College, University of Coimbra, Coimbra, Portugal

5 Polytechnic Institute of Coimbra, ESTESC-Coimbra Health School, Ciências Biomédicas Laboratoriais, Coimbra, Portugal

*Address all correspondence to: asmonteiro@fcsaude.ubi.pt

References

[1] Lassmann H, Brück W, Lucchinetti CF. The immunopathology of multiple sclerosis: An overview. In: Brain Pathology. 2007. p. 210-218. DOI: 10.1111/j.1750-3639.2007.00064.x

[2] Noseworthy JH, Lucchinetti C, Rodriguez M W, BG. Multiple Sclerosis. N Engl J Med. 2000;343:938-952. DOI: 10.1056/NEJM200009283431307

[3] Goverman J. Autoimmune T cell responses in the central nervous system. Nat Rev. Immunol. 2009;9(6):393. Doi:10.1038/nri2550

[4] Haji Abdolvahab M, Mofrad MRK, Schellekens H. Interferon Beta: From molecular level to therapeutic effects. Vol. 326, international review of cell and molecular biology. Elsevier Inc.; 2016. 343-372 p. DOI: 10.1016/bs.ircmb.2016.06.001

[5] Dhib-Jalbut S, Marks S. Interferon-β mechanisms of action in multiple sclerosis. Neurology. 2010;74(SUPPL.). DOI: 10.1212/WNL.0b013e3181c97d99

[6] Ziemssen T, Akgün K, Brück W. Molecular biomarkers in multiple sclerosis. J Neuroinflammation. 2019;16(1):1-11. DOI: 10.1186/s12974-019-1674-2

[7] Hauser SL, Oksenberg JR. The Neurobiology of Multiple Sclerosis: Genes, Inflammation, and Neurodegeneration. 2006;61-76. DOI: 10.1016/j.neuron.2006.09.011

[8] Kamm CP, Uitdehaag M, Polman CH. Neuro-Update: Multiple Sclerosis Multiple Sclerosis: Current Knowledge. 2014;132-141. DOI: 10.1159/000360528

[9] Dendrou CA, Fugger L, Friese MA. Immunopathology of multiple sclerosis. Vol. 15, nature reviews immunology. Nature Publishing Group; 2015. p. 545-558. DOI: 10.1038/nri3871

[10] Comabella M, Khoury SJ. Immunopathogenesis of multiple sclerosis. Clin Immunol. 2012;142(1):2-8. DOI: 10.1016/j.clim.2011.03.004

[11] Vaughn CB, Jakimovski D, Kavak KS, Ramanathan M, Benedict RHB, Zivadinov R, et al. Epidemiology and treatment of multiple sclerosis in elderly populations. Vol. 15, Nature Reviews Neurology. Springer US; 2019. p. 329-42. DOI: 10.1038/s41582-019-0183-3

[12] Simmons SB, Pierson ER, Lee SY, Goverman JM. Modeling the heterogeneity of multiple sclerosis in animals. Vol. 34, Trends in Immunology. 2013. p. 410-422. DOI: 10.1016/j.it.2013.04.006

[13] Thompson AJ, Baranzini SE, Geurts J, Hemmer B, Ciccarelli O. Multiple sclerosis. Lancet. 2018;391(10130):1622-1636. DOI: 10.1016/S0140-6736(18)30481-1

[14] Jones AP, Kermode AG, Lucas RM, Carroll WM, Nolan D, Hart PH. Circulating immune cells in multiple sclerosis. Vol. 187, clinical and experimental immunology. Blackwell Publishing Ltd.; 2017. p. 193-203. DOI: 10.1111/cei.12878

[15] Hegen H, Auer M, Deisenhammer F. Pharmacokinetic considerations in the treatment of multiple sclerosis with interferon-β. Vol. 11, Expert Opinion on Drug Metabolism and Toxicology. 2015. p. 1803-1819. DOI: 10.1517/17425255.2015.1094055

[16] Rizzo F, Giacomini E, Mechelli R, Buscarinu MC, Salvetti M, Severa M, et al. Interferon-β therapy specifically reduces pathogenic memory B cells in multiple sclerosis patients by inducing a FAS-mediated apoptosis. Immunol Cell Biol. 2016 Oct 1;94(9):886-894. DOI: 10.1038/icb.2016.55

[17] Dendrou CA, Fugger L. ScienceDirect Immunomodulation in multiple sclerosis: promises and pitfalls. Curr Opin Immunol. 2017;49:37-43. DOI: 10.1016/j.coi.2017.08.013

[18] Mendes A, Sá MJ. Classical immunomodulatory therapy in multiple sclerosis: How it acts, how it works. Arq Neuropsiquiatr. 2011;69(3):536-543. DOI: 10.1590/S0004-282X20 11000400024

[19] Axtell RC, Raman C, Steinman L. Type i interferons: Beneficial in Th1 and detrimental in Th17 autoimmunity. Vol. 44, Clinical Reviews in Allergy and Immunology. 2013. p. 114-120. DOI: 10.1007/s12016-011-8296-5

[20] Baufeld C, O'Loughlin E, Calcagno N, Madore C, Butovsky O. differential contribution of microglia and monocytes in neurodegenerative diseases. Vol. 125, Journal of Neural Transmission. Springer Vienna; 2018. p. 809-826. DOI: 10.1007/s00702-017-1795-7

[21] Wong KL, Yeap WH, Tai JJY, Ong SM, Dang TM, Wong SC. The three human monocyte subsets: Implications for health and disease. Immunol Res. 2012;53(1-3):41-57. DOI: 10.1007/s12026-012-8297-3

[22] Kasper LH, Reder AT. Immunomodulatory activity of interferon-beta. Vol. 1, Annals of Clinical and Translational Neurology. 2014. p. 622-631. DOI: 10.1002/acn3.84

[23] Severa M, Rizzo F, Giacomini E, Salvetti M, Coccia EM. IFN-β and multiple sclerosis: Cross-talking of immune cells and integration of immunoregulatory networks. Cytokine Growth Factor Rev. 2015;26(2):229-239. DOI: 10.1016/j.cytogfr.2014.11.005

[24] Waschbisch A, Schröder S, Schraudner D, Sammet L, Weksler B, Melms A, et al. Pivotal role for CD16 + monocytes in immune surveillance of the central nervous system. J Immunol. 2016;196(4):1558-1567. DOI: 10.4049/jimmunol.1501960

[25] Boltjes A, van Wijk F. Human dendritic cell functional specialization in steady-state and inflammation. Front Immunol. 2014;5(APR):1-13. DOI: 10.3389/fimmu.2014.00131

[26] Pennel L, Fisher E. IFN-β effects on dendritic cells in EAE. Immunology. 2016;38(1):42-49. DOI: 10.1111/imm.12781

[27] Monteiro A, Rosado P, Rosado L, Fonseca AM, Coucelo M, Paiva A. Alterations in peripheral blood monocyte and dendritic cell subset homeostasis in relapsing–remitting multiple sclerosis patients. J Neuroimmunol. 2021;350(September 2020):577433. DOI: 10.1016/j.jneuroim.2020.577433

[28] Bergh FT, Dayyani F, Ziegler-heitbrock L. Impact of type-I-interferon on monocyte subsets and their differentiation to dendritic cells An in vivo and ex vivo study in multiple sclerosis patients treated with interferon-beta. 2004;146:176-188. DOI: 10.1016/j.neuroim.2003.10.037

[29] Ziegler-Heitbrock L. Blood monocytes and their subsets: Established features and open questions. Front Immunol. 2015;6(AUG):1-5. DOI: 10.3389/fimmu.2015.00423

[30] Zang YC, Skinner SM, Robinson RR, Li S, Rivera VM, Hutton GJ, et al. Regulation of differentiation and functional properties of monocytes and monocyte-derived dendritic cells by interferon beta in multiple sclerosis. Mult Scler. 2004;10(5):499-506. DOI: 10.1191/135245804ms1081oa

[31] Kantor AB, Deng J, Waubant E, Lin H, Becker CH, Lacy JR, et al.

Identification of short-term pharmacodynamic effects of interferon-beta-1a in multiple sclerosis subjects with broad- based phenotypic profiling. J Neuroimmunol. 2007;188(1-2):103-116. DOI: 10.1016/j.jneuroim.2007.05.009

[32] Marckmann S, Wiesemann E, Hilse R, Trebst C, Stangel M. Interferon-b up-regulates the expression of co-stimulatory molecules CD80, CD86 and CD40 on monocytes: significance for treatment of multiple sclerosis. 2004;499-506. DOI: 10.1111/j.1365-2249.2004.02624.x

[33] Kunkl M, Frascolla S, Amormino C, Volpe E, Tuosto L. T Helper cells: The modulators of inflammation in Multiple Sclerosis. Cells. 2020;9(2):1-20. DOI: 10.1191/1352458504ms1081oa

[34] Machado-Santos J, Saji E, Tröscher AR, Paunovic M, Liblau R, Gabriely G, et al. The compartmentalized inflammatory response in the multiple sclerosis brain is composed of tissue-resident CD8+ T lymphocytes and B cells. Brain. 2018 Jul 1;141(7):2066-2082. DOI: 10.1093/brain/awy151

[35] Kaskow BJ, Baecher-allan C. Effector T cells in Multiple Sclerosis. Cold Spring Harbor Perspectives in Medicine 2018;1-14. DOI: 10.1101/cshperspect.a029025

[36] Peelen E, Thewissen M, Knippenberg S, Smolders J, Muris AH, Menheere P, et al. Fraction of IL-10+ and IL-17+ CD8 T cells is increased in MS patients in remission and during a relapse, but is not influenced by immune modulators. J Neuroimmunol. 2013;258 DOI: 10.1016/j.jneuroim.2013.02.014

[37] Stadhouders R, Lubberts E, Hendriks RW. A cellular and molecular view of T helper 17 cell plasticity in autoimmunity. J Autoimmun. 2018;87:1-15. DOI: 10.1016/j.jaut.2017.12.007

[38] Cipollini V, Anrather J, Orzi F, Iadecola C. Th17 and Cognitive Impairment: Possible Mechanisms of Action. 2019;13(November):1-12. DOI: 10.3389/fnana.2019.00095

[39] Sie C, Korn T, Mitsdoerffer M. Th17 cells in central nervous system autoimmunity. Exp Neurol. 2014;262(Part A):18-27. DOI: 10.1016/j.expneurol.2014.03.009

[40] Li YF, Zhang SX, Ma XW, Xue YL, Gao C, Li XY. Levels of peripheral Th17 cells and serum Th17-related cytokines in patients with multiple sclerosis: A meta-analysis. Mult Scler Relat Disord. 2017;18:20-25. DOI: 10.1016/j.msard.2017.09.003

[41] Monteiro A, Rosado P, Rosado L, Fonseca AM, Paiva A. Alterations in circulating T cell functional subpopulations in interferon-beta treated multiple sclerosis patients: A pilot study. J Neuroimmunol. 2020;339. DOI: 10.1016/j.jneuroim.2019.577113

[42] Rodrigues G, Passos D, Sato DK, Becker J, Fujihara K. Th17 cells pathways in Multiple Sclerosis and Neuromyelitis Optica Spectrum disorders: Pathophysiological and therapeutic implications. Hindawi. 2016;2016. DOI: 10.1155/2016/5314541

[43] Van Langelaar J, Van Der Vuurst De Vries RM, Janssen M, Wierenga-wolf AF, spilt IM, Siepman TA, et al. T helper 17.1 cells associate with multiple sclerosis disease activity: Perspectives for early intervention. Brain. 2018;141(5):1334-1349. DOI: 10.1093/brain/awy069

[44] Raphael I, Nalawade S, Eagar TN, Forsthuber TG. Cytokine T cell subsets and their signature cytokines in autoimmune and inflammatory diseases. Cytokine. 2014. DOI: 10.1016/j.cyto.2014.09.011

[45] Libera DD, Di Mitri D, Bergami A, Centonze D, Gasperini C, Grasso MG,

et al. T regulatory cells are markers of disease activity in multiple sclerosis patients. PLoS One. 2011;6(6). DOI: 10.1371/journal.pone.0021386

[46] Haas J, Fritzsching B, Trübswetter P, Korporal M, Milkova L, Fritz B, et al. Prevalence of Newly Generated Naive Regulatory T Cells (T reg) Is Critical for T reg Suppressive Function and Determines T reg Dysfunction in Multiple Sclerosis. J Immunol. 2007;179(2):1322-1330. DOI: 10.4049/jimmunol.179.2.1322

[47] Venken K, Hellings N, Broekmans T, Hensen K, Rummens J, Stinissen P. Natural naive CD4 + CD25 + CD127 low regulatory T cell (Treg) development and function are disturbed in Multiple Sclerosis patients: Recovery of memory Treg homeostasis during disease progression. J Immunol. 2008;180(9):6411-6420. DOI: 10.4049/jimmunol.180.9.6411

[48] Scherm MG, Ott VB, Daniel C. Follicular helper T cells in autoimmunity. Curr Diab Rep. 2016;16(8). DOI: 10.1007/s11892-016-0770-2

[49] Quinn JL, Axtell RC. Emerging role of follicular T helper cells in multiple sclerosis and experimental autoimmune encephalomyelitis. Int J Mol Sci. 2018;19(10). DOI: 10.3390/ijms19103233

[50] Song W, Craft J. T follicular helper cell heterogeneity: Time, space, and function. Vol. 288, Immunological Reviews. 2019. p. 85-96. DOI: 10.1111/imr.12740

[51] Romme Christensen J, Börnsen L, Ratzer R, Piehl F, Khademi M, Olsson T, et al. Systemic inflammation in progressive multiple sclerosis involves follicular T-helper, Th17- and activated B-cells and correlates with progression. PLoS One. 2013 Jan [cited 2015 Jan 12];8(3):e57820. DOI: 10.1371/journal.pone.0057820

[52] Prinz I, Silva-Santos B, Pennington DJ. Functional development of γδ T cells. Eur J Immunol. 2013;43(8):1988-1994. DOI: 10.1002/eji.201343759

[53] Serre K, Silva-Santos B. Molecular mechanisms of differentiation of murine pro-inflammatory γδ T cell subsets. Front Immunol. 2013;4(DEC):1-7. DOI: 10.3389/fimmu.2013.00431

[54] Battistini L, Caccamo N, Borsellino G, Meraviglia S, Angelini DF, Dieli F, et al. Homing and memory patterns of human γδ T cells in physiopathological situations. Vol. 7, Microbes and Infection. 2005. p. 510-517. DOI: 10.1016/j.micinf.2004.12.008

[55] Blink SE, Miller SD. The contribution of gammadelta T cells to the pathogenesis of EAE and MS. Curr Mol Med. 2009;9(1):15-22. DOI: 10.2174/156652409787314516

[56] Monteiro A, Cruto C, Rosado P, Martinho A, Rosado L, Fonseca M, et al. Characterization of circulating gamma-delta T cells in relapsing vs. remission multiple sclerosis. J Neuroimmunol. 2018;318. DOI: 10.1016/j.jneuroim.2018.02.009

[57] Iarlori C, Reale M, Lugaresi A, De Luca G, Bonanni L, Di Iorio A, et al. RANTES production and expression is reduced in relapsing–remitting multiple sclerosis patients treated with interferon-β-1b. J Neuroimmunol. 2000;107(1):100-107. DOI: 10.1016/S0165-5728(00)00261-7

[58] Szczuciński A, Losy J. Chemokines and chemokine receptors in multiple sclerosis. Potential targets for new therapies. Acta Neurol Scand. 2007;115(3):137-146. DOI: 10.1111/j.1600-0404.2006.00749.x

[59] Lehmann-Horn K, Kronsbein HC, Weber MS. Targeting B cells in the

treatment of multiple sclerosis: Recent advances and remaining challenges. Ther Adv Neurol Disord. 2013 May [cited 2015 Jan 10];6(3):161-173. DOI: 10.1177/1756285612474333

[60] Michel L, Touil H, Pikor NB, Gommerman JL, Prat A, Bar-Or A. B Cells in the multiple sclerosis central nervous system: Trafficking and contribution to CNS-compartmentalized inflammation. Vol. 6, Frontiers in immunology. Frontiers Media S.a.; 2015. DOI: 10.3389/fimmu.2015.00636

[61] Sospedra M. B cells in multiple sclerosis. Vol. 31, Current Opinion in Neurology. Lippincott Williams and Wilkins; 2018. p. 256-262. DOI: 10.1097/WCO.0000000000000563

[62] Li R, Patterson KR, Bar-Or A. Reassessing B Cell contributions in multiple sclerosis. Vol. 19, nature immunology. Nature Publishing Group; 2018. p. 696-707. DOI: 10.1038/s41590-018-0135-x

[63] Perez-Andres M, Paiva B, Nieto WG, Caraux a., Schmitz a., Almeida J, et al. Human peripheral blood B-Cell compartments: A crossroad in B-cell traffic. Cytom Part B - Clin Cytom. 2010 Jan [cited 2014 Nov 5];78(SUPPL. 1):S47-60. DOI: 10.1002/cyto.b.20547

[64] Schubert RD, Hu Y, Kumar G, Szeto S, Abraham P, Winderl J, et al. IFN-β treatment requires B cells for efficacy in Neuroautoimmunity. J Immunol. 2015 Mar 1;194(5):2110-2116. DOI: 10.4049/jimmunol.1402029

[65] Longbrake EE, Cross AH. Effect of multiple sclerosis disease-modifying therapies on b cells and humoral immunity. Vol. 73, JAMA neurology. American Medical Association; 2016. p. 219-225. DOI: 10.1001/jamaneurol.2015.3977

[66] Monteiro A, Cruto C, Rosado P, Rosado L, Fonseca AM, Paiva A. Interferon-beta treated-multiple sclerosis patients exhibit a decreased ratio between immature/transitional B cell subset and plasmablasts. J Neuroimmunol. 2019;326. DOI: 10.1016/j.jneuroim.2018.11.001

[67] Mitsdoerffer M, Peters a. tertiary lymphoid organs in central nervous system autoimmunity. Vol. 7, Frontiers in immunology. Frontiers Media S.a.; 2016. DOI: 10.3389/fimmu.2016.00451

[68] Kieseier BC. The mechanism of action of interferon-beta in relapsing multiple sclerosis. CNS Drugs. 2011;25(6):491-502. DOI: 10.2165/11591110-000000000-00000

Chapter 5

Amino Acids as Neurotransmitters. The Balance between Excitation and Inhibition as a Background for Future Clinical Applications

Yaroslav R. Nartsissov

Abstract

For more than 30 years, amino acids have been well-known (and essential) participants in neurotransmission. They act as both neuromediators and metabolites in nervous tissue. Glycine and glutamic acid (glutamate) are prominent examples. These amino acids are agonists of inhibitory and excitatory membrane receptors, respectively. Moreover, they play essential roles in metabolic pathways and energy transformation in neurons and astrocytes. Despite their obvious effects on the brain, their potential role in therapeutic methods remains uncertain in clinical practice. In the current chapter, a comparison of the crosstalk between these two systems, which are responsible for excitation and inhibition in neurons, is presented. The interactions are discussed at the metabolic, receptor, and transport levels. Reaction-diffusion and a convectional flow into the interstitial fluid create a balanced distribution of glycine and glutamate. Indeed, the neurons' final physiological state is a result of a balance between the excitatory and inhibitory influences. However, changes to the glycine and/or glutamate pools under pathological conditions can alter the state of nervous tissue. Thus, new therapies for various diseases may be developed on the basis of amino acid medication.

Keywords: glycine, glutamate, neurotransmission

1. Introduction

Even for students just beginning to study biochemistry and physiology, it is immediately apparent that amino acids (AAs) are among the most important molecules in nature. Their functions are broad and varied. Indeed, protein synthesis relies on the well-known polymerization of AAs to form a peptide bond. This property is the most famous aspect of AAs. However, many AAs have specific individual functions, such as neurotransmission [1], cellular energy metabolism [2], and detoxification [3, 4]. Accumulating evidence in recent years has demonstrated that AAs also regulate both the expression of genes and the protein phosphorylation cascade. Moreover, hormones and different low-molecular-weight biologically important chemical compounds can be synthesized from AAs [5]. AAs can be divided into essential and nonessential categories. If the body cannot synthesize the carbon skeleton of an amino acid, then it is considered nutritionally essential.

Indeed, the diet must contain such AAs. The dietary essentiality of other AAs (e.g., arginine, glycine, proline, and taurine) is determined by the developmental stage and species [6]. In contrast, if AAs can be synthesized de novo in a species-dependent manner, they are considered nonessential. Accumulating evidence has led to the concept of functional AAs (FAAs), which are defined as AAs that regulate key metabolic pathways to improve the health, survival, growth, development, lactation, and reproduction of organisms [7]. Since the late 1970s, researchers have generally agreed that amino acids can also function as inhibitory or excitatory neurotransmitters [8]. It should be noted that in neurochemistry, the term "neurotransmitter" is usually used synonymously with "neuromediator," another term for a chemical participant in connections between neurons and neuroglia cells. Because these terms are exchangeable, they will both be used in the text. Based on their effects on vertebrate nerve cells, γ-aminobutyric acid (GABA), glycine, and taurine fall into the class of inhibitory amino acids, whereas glutamate and aspartate fall into the class of excitatory compounds [9]. Indeed, GABA is considered the main inhibitory neurotransmitter in the central nervous system (CNS) [10], but it is not truly a member of the AA family. Although taurine also plays a role in inhibitory neuromediation [11] and serves as an osmoeffector to regulate volume in astrocytes [12], this compound is considered a derivative of cysteine, and, similar to GABA, not a true amino acid. Thus, the remaining excitatory/inhibitory amino acid neurotransmitters are glutamate, aspartate, and glycine. The first and third are the most prominent members of the AA family. The processes that regulate glutamate and glycine in the CNS are (i) transportation, (ii) biochemical transformations in metabolic pathways, and (iii) interactions with membrane receptors. In the current chapter, the crosstalk between the processes mentioned above for both glutamate and glycine is presented because the final state of neurons seems to be a result of the balance between these excitatory and inhibitory influences.

2. The membrane transport system of amino acids

Glutamate and glycine are nonessential amino acids; their levels differ depending on the location. The extracellular glutamate concentration around quiescent neurons is less than 1 μM, while its concentration in the cytoplasm is much higher, at approximately 2 mM [13]. The brain sequesters glycine in concentrations of 600 μM [14], with a basal concentration in the cerebrospinal fluid (CSF) of ~6 μM [15], compared to a plasma concentration of ~250 μM [16]. Because no extracellular enzymes degrade glutamate and glycine, maintaining these low extracellular concentrations requires cellular uptake of both compounds. Thus, the activity of the carriers directly regulates receptor response to neuron activation. Indeed, glutamate and glycine serve as neuromediators in the extracellular fluid because the binding site of AA receptors is exposed to the outer surface of cells. Consequently, the release of AA into the extracellular fluid controls receptor activation and active states are controlled by the removal of AAs from the extracellular fluid [17]. This uptake is catalyzed by a family of transporter proteins located on the cell surface of both astrocytes and neurons [17]. A high-affinity glutamatergic uptake system was observed in the mammalian brain in the 1970s. Subsequently, excitatory amino acid transporters (EAATs) were experimentally identified. They transport glutamate and aspartate across the plasma membrane. Notably, EAATs are part of the well-known solute carrier 1 (SLC1) family of transmembrane amino acid transporters [18]. Thus, released glutamate molecules can be removed from the synaptic cleft by the brain transporters; this process will initiate the glutamate-glutamine cycle, eventually restoring the pool of the neuromediator in synaptic vesicles [19]. Five EAAT isoforms, human EAAT1-5, have been identified; they correspond to GLAST1/GLT-1/EAAC1/EAAT4/EAAT5 in rodents, respectively [20]. In addition, the EAAT4 and EAAT5 subtypes were identified, with EAAT5 predominantly expressed in the retina. Notably, the transport cycle times of EAATs are relatively slow and their high affinity for glutamate makes it possible to sequester low glutamate concentrations from the extracellular space, preventing excitotoxicity. The slow transportation rate may in part be overcome by rapid surface diffusion and transporter tracking of EAATs upon glutamate stimulation [21]. The SLC1 family also contains two neutral amino acid transporters, alanine serine cysteine transporters 1 and 2 (ASCT1 and 2), which share high sequence homology with the EAATs [22]. EAAT1 and EAAT2 are glutamate transporters that are mostly expressed in astrocytes. These two glutamate transporters are responsible for most of the glutamate clearance in the brain. EAAT2 is widely expressed in the cerebral cortex and the hippocampus [13]. Moreover, GLT-1/EAAT2 accounts for approximately 90% of the total glutamate uptake in the brain, and thus, it is considered the most important glutamate transporter subtype in the CNS. This transporter is predominantly but not exclusively expressed in astrocytes [22]. Glutamate transporters couple glutamate uptake to the transport of inorganic ions. It is now generally accepted that 3 Na^+ ions and 1 H^+ ion are cotransported and 1 K^+ ion is counter-transported with the uptake of each glutamate molecule. Based on this stoichiometry, glutamate transporters were calculated to concentrate glutamate up to 5×10^6-fold inside cells under physiological conditions. This glutamate transport is electrogenic [23].

The extracellular levels of glycine in inhibitory and excitatory synapses are controlled by glycine transporters (GlyTs). Both subtypes, GlyT1 and GlyT2, belong

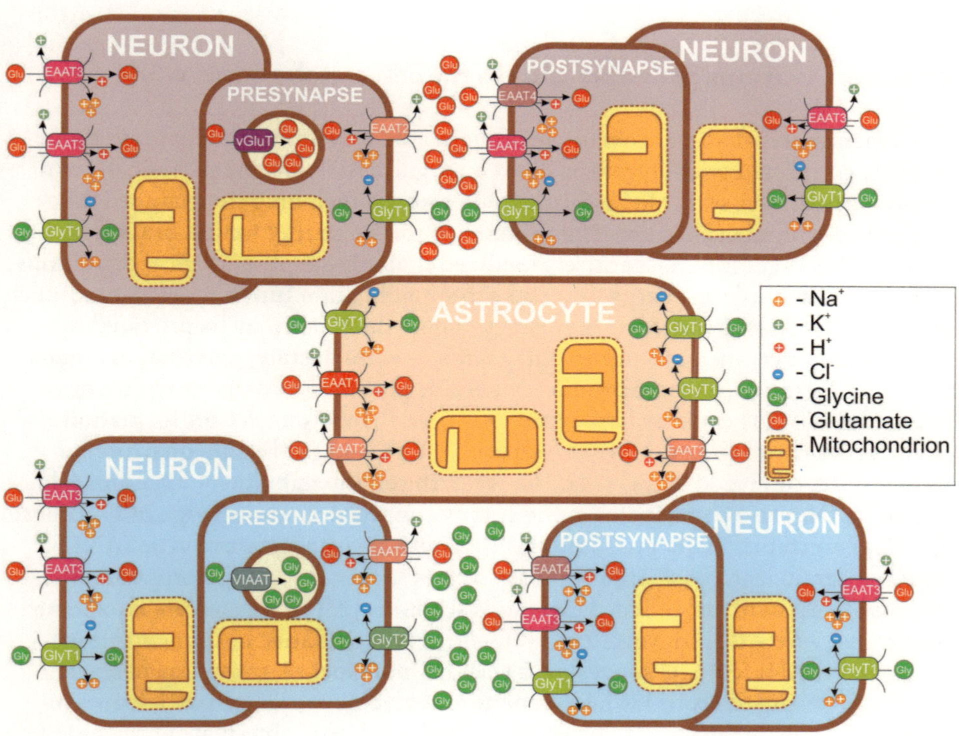

Figure 1.
Membrane carriers are responsible for clearance of glutamate/glycine from interstitial fluid (ISF) in the CNS. The scheme indicates two types of neurons. Some are excitatory and glutamatergic (the upper part of the scheme). Other neurons are inhibitory and glycinergic (the lower part of the scheme). Both types of neurons are interconnected with astrocytes. Moreover, glycine and glutamate are accessible for both types of cells. AA transporters (EAAT, GlyT, etc.) are found in all cell membranes but have differing isoenzyme compositions.

to the sodium-dependent solute carrier 6 (SLC6) family of transporters, but they have different regional and cellular expression patterns in the CNS, different stoichiometries (that is, different numbers of sodium ions that are co-transported with every glycine molecule) and varying abilities to reverse-transport glycine into the extracellular space. To date, five variants of GlyT1 (GlyT1a, GlyT1b, GlyT1c, GlyT1d, and GlyT1e) and three variants of GlyT2 (GlyT2a, GlyT2b, and GlyT2c) have been identified and occur as a result of alternative promoter usage and/or splicing, but the relative distributions of these within the CNS have not been fully characterized [21].

The essential function of membrane transporters is to accumulate neuromediators in vesicles. At presynaptic terminals, vesicular glutamate transporters (vGluTs; SLC17A7, -6, and -8) load glutamate into synaptic vesicles. The two subtypes of vGluTs, vGluT1, and vGluT2, are expressed in excitatory neurons in a complementary manner in the brain, composing two subsets of excitatory neurons [13]. Glycine also actively accumulates in synaptic vesicles through vesicular inhibitory amino acid transporter (VIAAT); currently, only one type of transporter (SLC32A1) is known to be responsible for this process [18]. The scheme of balanced neuromediator transport is represented in **Figure 1**.

Remarkably, both glutamate and glycine transporters have mechanisms that include sodium ion transport. This means that neuromediator uptake is accompanied by changes in membrane potential. Moreover, the intake of both glutamate and glycine initiates several metabolic reactions in neurons and astrocytes. However, these reactions are spatially distributed, and the fate of the neuromediators is functionally determined by different cells. Interestingly, the metabolic transformations of AAs are closely related to ATP production by mitochondria and the oxidation of glucose.

3. Transformations of amino acids in the cell metabolic network

As mentioned above, any example of metabolic transformation in brain tissue is tightly connected with glycolysis Therefore, glutamate/glycine participation in metabolic pathways seems to be considered correctly including the main neighbor reactions of glucose oxidation. The primary source of energy for the brain is glucose. This sugar is almost entirely oxidized under basal physiological conditions, providing nearly all the energy necessary to support brain function. However, when supplemental energy is needed, necessary energy demands may be provided by other metabolites, such as ketones, fatty acids, acetate, lactate, and certain amino acids [19]. Pyruvate, the end product of aerobic glycolysis, can enter the tricarboxylic acid (TCA) cycle by two different routes: (1) via acetyl-CoA formation, catalyzed by the pyruvate dehydrogenase complex, and (2) by the formation of oxaloacetate, catalyzed by PC [24]. However, the end metabolite of anaerobic glycolysis, lactate, also participates in the energy supply of neurons (**Figure 2**). Pellerin and Magistretti originally proposed the astrocyte-neuron lactate shuttle (ANLS) model, wherein lactate released from astrocytes serves as a buffer compound in response to a glutamate-induced glycolysis stimulus [25]. Then, lactate is exported to neurons, where it is converted to pyruvate to fuel oxidative phosphorylation.

Thus, the ANLS model suggests that lactate, not glucose, provides energetic support for firing neurons [26]. Glutamate and glycine are active participants in these metabolic processes. Exclusion of most blood-borne glutamate at the blood-brain barrier (BBB) and a net removal of glutamine from the brain indicate that the cerebral pools of glutamate are largely produced within the brain [27]. The stability of glutamate concentration is maintained by two main reactions. Glutamine synthetase (GS), which is found in astrocytes, is the only known enzyme to date that is capable of a reversible conversion between glutamine and glutamate and

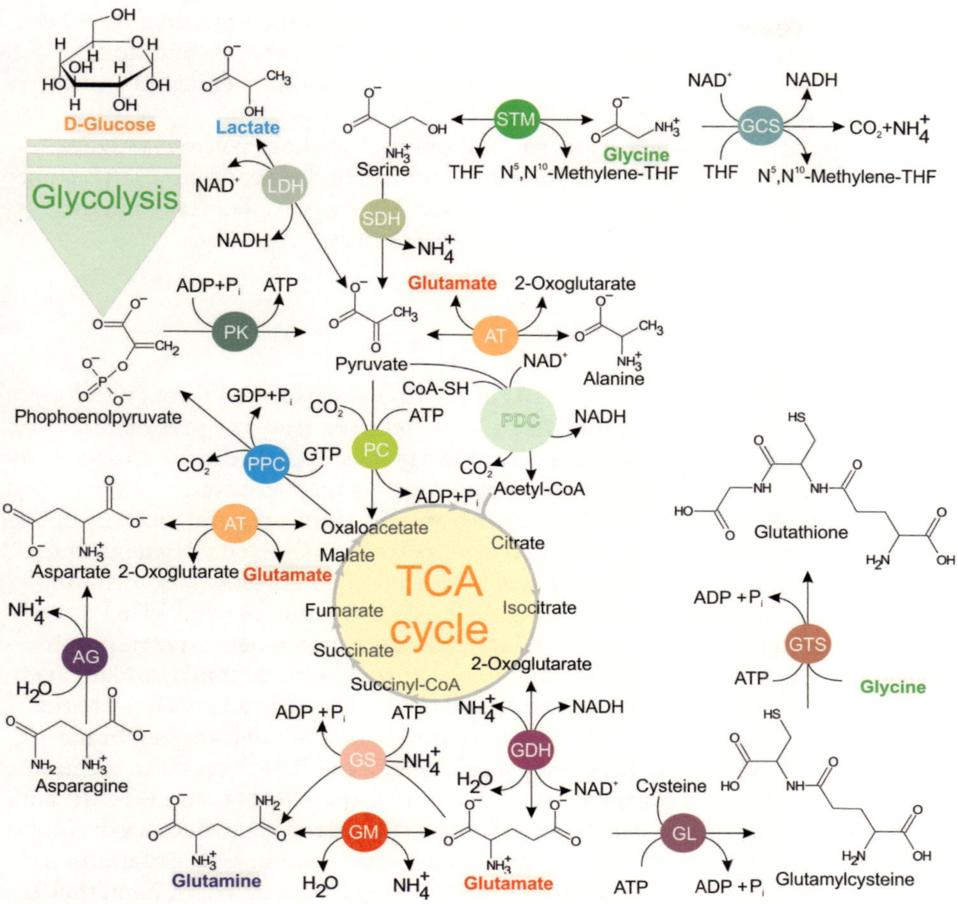

Figure 2.
A scheme of the metabolic pathways involved in general glutamate/glycine transformations. The reactions occur in various intracellular localizations and can be duplicated in different compartments. The main metabolic pathways (glycolysis and the tricarboxylic acid (TCA) cycle) are labeled. The enzyme abbreviations are as follows: GM: glutaminase; GS: glutamine synthetase; GDH: glutamate dehydrogenase; GL: glutamylcysteine ligase; GTS: glutathione synthetase; AG: asparaginase; AT: aminotransferase; PPC: phosphoenolpyruvate carboxykinase; PC: pyruvate carboxylase; PDC: pyruvate dehydrogenase complex; PK: pyruvate kinase; LDH: lactate dehydrogenase; SDH: serine dehydrogenase; STM: serine transhydroxymethylase; and GCS: the glycine cleavage system. Other abbreviations are as follows: NAD+: Nicotinamide adenine dinucleotide (oxidized); NADH: Nicotinamide adenine dinucleotide (reduced); ATP: Adenosine triphosphate; ADP: Adenosine diphosphate; and THF:Tetrahydrofolate.

ammonia in the mammalian brain [28]. Furthermore, cells can convert glutamate to glutamine in an ATP-dependent process catalyzed by glutamine synthetase. Astrocytic uptake of glutamate and release of glutamine, together with neuronal uptake of glutamine and release of glutamate, constitute the glutamate-glutamine cycle [29]. However, much of the glutamate taken up by astrocytes is destined for oxidative degradation, which first requires conversion to the TCA cycle intermediate 2-oxoglutarate. This can take place via transamination by aminotransferase (AT) or via oxidative deamination by glutamate dehydrogenase (GDH) [30].

Once glycine passes into a cell by uptake by GlyTs, the intracellular glycine concentration can be regulated via synthesis from L-serine within the cell, which itself can be synthesized from glycolysis intermediates and L-glutamate [24]. The major pathway for the glycine catabolism involves the oxidative cleavage of glycine to CO2, NH^{4+}, and a methylene group (–CH2–), which is accepted by tetrahydrofolate (H^4folate) in a reversible reaction catalyzed by the glycine cleavage system (also called glycine synthase) [31]. The glycine cleavage system is essentially reversible but catalyzes glycine synthesis significantly only under anaerobic conditions, such as in anaerobic bacteria or anaerobic systems in vitro supplemented with $NADH+H^+$ [32].

Taken together, all known information about the metabolic pathways suggests that glutamate and glycine self-regulate the processes of their concentration restoration and mutual transformation. Additionally, oxidative phosphorylation in the mitochondria also plays a key role in the balance of these AAs.

4. CNS receptors of amino acids

The neuromediator function of AAs in the CNS is performed through the activation of membrane receptors. After being released from the presynaptic membrane into a synaptic cleft, glutamate and glycine rapidly diffuse to a postsynaptic membrane, where appropriate receptors are further activated.

Glutamate receptors are divided into two groups: ionotropic glutamate receptors (iGluRs) and metabotropic glutamate receptors (mGluRs). Excitatory neurotransmission throughout the CNS is mediated by ligand-gated ion channels, including ionotropic glutamate receptors (iGluRs) [33]. Abnormalities in iGluRs lead to a wide range of neurological diseases. Glutamate, the primary neurotransmitter in almost all synapses in the CNS, is released from presynaptic terminals and diffuses to the postsynaptic membrane, where it binds to iGluRs. This process leads to the opening of ion channels, allowing cations to flow in. Thus, the transmembrane channel rapidly depolarizes the postsynaptic membrane. The decrease in membrane potential initiates signal transduction in the postsynaptic neuron. In the iGluR family, four subtypes of integral membrane proteins have been identified in vertebrates based on their pharmacological properties and sequence homologies: α-amino-3-hydroxy-5-methyl-4-isoxazolepropionic acid (AMPA), kainate (KA), N-methyl-D-aspartate (NMDA), and δ-receptors [34]. Subsequent cloning studies have revealed that NMDARs are assembled as heteromers that differ in subunit composition. To date, seven different subunits have been identified and categorized into three subfamilies according to sequence homology [35]. Each iGluR family member exhibits specific kinetic and pharmacological properties in addition to playing a unique role in neurotransmission [36]. The iGluRs are ligand-gated ion channels that are permeable to Na^+ and K^+ (and Ca^{2+} in some instances), whereas the mGluRs are G protein-coupled receptors that trigger second messenger cascades. The early component and the late component of neurotransmission are assumed to be mediated by AMPARs and NMDARs/KARs, respectively. This assumption is based on receptor kinetics, as AMPARs are faster and NMDARs/KARs are slower. Nevertheless, acoustic signals are transferred by all of these iGluRs in a precise and reliable manner. Moreover, some auditory processing neurons have a fourth type of iGluR, the delta receptor [34]. The open, or conducting, conformation of the iGluR ion channel is nonselective for monovalent cations. Membrane excitation is often driven by channel permeability to Ca^{2+}. This Ca^{2+} influx and its physiological and pathological consequences depend strongly on the specific iGluR subtype and the specific subunits in its oligomeric complex [37].

mGluRs are G protein-coupled receptors (GPCRs) that, following activation, regulate both G protein-dependent and G protein-independent signalling pathways. According to sequence homology, cell signalling activation, and agonist selectivity, the mGluRs have been divided into eight subtypes (from mGlu1 to mGlu8). These subtypes comprise three different subgroups (from I to III) [38]. Group I mGluRs (mGlu1 and mGlu5) are functionally linked to polyphosphoinositide (PI) hydrolysis

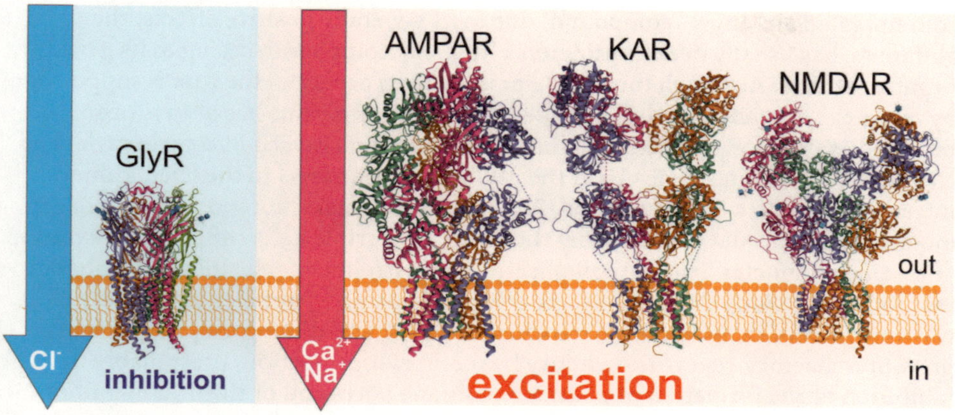

Figure 3.
A reconstruction of possible AA ionotropic receptors in the CNS. The images were created using the data collected in the Protein Data Bank (PDB) (https://www.rcsb.org/). The scaled images show GlyR (6UBS, Danio rerio, [44]), AMPAR (5IDE, Rattus norvegicus, [45]), KAR (6KZM, Rattus norvegicus, [46]) and NMDAR (7EOQ, Homo sapiens, [47]).

and are negatively coupled with K^+ channels. Both group II (mGlu2 and mGlu3) and group III (mGlu4, mGlu6, mGlu7, and mGlu8) mGluRs negatively regulate adenylate cyclase and activate mitogen-activated protein kinase (MAPK) and PI-3-kinase pathways [39]. mGluRs are usually localized on synaptic and extrasynaptic membranes in both glia and neurons. Group I mGluRs are generally postsynaptic, surrounding ionotropic receptors, and modulate depolarization and synaptic excitability. Groups II and III are mostly expressed at the presynaptic level and control the release of neurotransmitters [39, 40]. mGluRs are heavily expressed throughout the basal ganglia (BG), where they modulate neuronal excitability, transmitter release, and long-term synaptic plasticity [41]. These receptors are coupled to different G proteins and modulate slow postsynaptic neuronal responses, either through presynaptic or postsynaptic machinery or through modulation of astrocyte function [42]. mGluRs are highly and diffusely expressed in glial cells. On the one hand, this increases the options for therapeutic interventions, but on the other hand, it makes it even more difficult to selectively target single receptors to yield neuroprotection (**Figure 3**) [43].

Glycine receptors (GlyRs), along with certain γ-aminobutyric acid receptors (GABAARs), are the principal determinants of fast inhibitory synaptic neurotransmission in the central nervous system (CNS). GlyR and GABAAR belong to the superfamily of pentameric ligand-gated ion channels (pLGICs) [33]. The two neurotransmitters (glycine and GABA) may be functionally interchangeable, and the multiple receptor subtypes with inhibitory influences provide diverse mechanisms for maintaining inhibitory homeostasis [35]. Inhibitory glycine receptors (GlyRs) are anion-selective ligand-gated ion channels (LGICs), which, together with GABAA receptors (GABAARs), nicotinic acetylcholine receptors (nAChRs), and serotonin type 3 receptors (5HT-3), form the eukaryotic Cys-loop family [36]. Several endogenous molecules, including neurotransmitters and neuromodulators (such as glutamate, Zn, and Ni), and exogenous substances, such as anaesthetics and alcohols, modulate GlyR function [40].

5. Participation in development of pathological processes

Despite their obvious physiological roles in protein synthesis, the cellular effects of glycine and glutamate in the CNS seem to be quite different. If glycine has been contemplated an "angel" compound, due to its generally positive effects, then glutamate has usually been considered a "demon" compound, owing to its generally negative effects. Although the last claim is far from accurate, the first is supported by many experimental findings. Indeed, the effect of glycine has always been reported as positive. It protects against oxidative stress caused by a wide variety of chemicals, drugs, and toxicants at the cellular or organ level in the liver, kidneys, intestines, and vascular system [34, 37]. Glycine is a major component of collagen molecules that is vital to stabilizing them to form a triple helix [48]. Administration of glycine attenuates diabetic complications in a streptozotocin-induced diabetic rat model [49]. Supplemental glycine effectively protects muscles in a variety of wasting models, including cancer cachexia, sepsis, and dieting [50]. Glycine may prevent ischaemia–reperfusion injury by direct cytoprotection, presumably by inhibition of the formation of plasma membrane pores and of the inflammatory response [38]. The cytoprotective and modulatory effects of glycine have been observed in many nonneuronal cell types. The action of glycine is mediated by classic or unconventional GlyRs, both inside and outside of the nervous system [51]. Glycine cytoprotection substantially overlaps with the number of agents that act on neuronal receptors with glycine as an agonist or coagonist. This observation has been confirmed by molecular pharmacology studies from multiple laboratories. The studies indicate highly constrained steric and conformational requirements for the interaction, which, along with the rapid on-off timing of the effects, is consistent with the involvement of reversible ligand-binding site interactions [52].

In contrast, glutamate is considered a toxic agent that yields excitotoxicity at overload concentrations. Indeed, the neurotoxic potential of glutamate has been recognized since the 1950s [53]. For example, a major driver of white matter demise is excitotoxicity, a consequence of the excessive glutamate released by vesicular and nonvesicular mechanisms from axons and glial cells. This excessive glutamate concentration results in overactivation of iGluRs profusely expressed by all cell compartments in white matter [54]. Generally, excitotoxicity involves a large inflow of Ca^{2+} and Na^{+} into neurons up to the conditions when Ca^{2+} concentrations reach critical levels, leading to cell injury or death [55]. Moreover, ambient extracellular glutamate is lower than the concentration known to trigger excitotoxicity and subsequent neurodegeneration; excitotoxicity is known to occur at extracellular glutamate concentrations as low as 2 to 5 μM, with swelling and apoptosis predominating at <20 μM glutamate and fast necrosis at >100 μM glutamate [56]. Excitotoxic neuronal death is involved in neurodegenerative diseases of the CNS, such as multiple sclerosis [57], Alzheimer's disease [58], Parkinson's disease [59], Huntington's disease [60], stroke, epilepsy, alcohol withdrawal, and amyotrophic lateral sclerosis [61]. However, the role of glutamate is not only excitotoxic. The assumption that neurodegenerative disease treatments should "fight against" glutamate is incorrect given the wrong function of glutamate in the CNS. As a part of normal physiological excitation, this AA must be properly regulated, but battling with glutamate receptors or the transport system will cause serious negative consequences. Instead, the level and functional activity of glutamate may be adjusted by metabolic processes, including glycine and oxidative phosphorylation, in mitochondria.

6. Balance is achieved through mutual interactions of the excitatory and inhibitory effects of amino acids

Because glutamate is the major mediator of excitatory signals as well as of nervous system plasticity, including cell elimination, it follows that glutamate needs to be present at the right concentrations in the right places at the right time [17].

These conditions are regulated by GS, GM, and EAATs and convectional diffusion in ISF. There is evidence that extracellular glutamate is not compartmentalized by EAATs under some conditions [62]. The most obvious shift in glutamate levels is observed under high GDH and AT activity. The general activation of bioenergetics decreases the excessive glutamate concentration by stimulating the TCA cycle. Moreover, glycine can participate in this shift in a variety of ways. GlyT-1 controls glycine release and reuptake, determines glycine availability at glycine binding sites on NMDA receptors [36] and coordinates neuronal-glial interactions at glutamatergic synapses [19]. Thus, glycine assists glutamate in the activation of astrocytes and further stimulates the mitochondria according to the ANLS hypothesis. Glycine can conjugate with glutamate in the GSH synthesis pathway (**Figure 1**). This mechanism is essential to maintain the redox status of neurons and to prevent oxidative stress and high levels of reactive oxygen species (ROS) synthesis. Neuronal mitochondria are the target of glutamate, which attenuates succinate dehydrogenase (a key enzyme of the TCA cycle) inhibition by oxaloacetate [63], with further induction of ROS production [64]. However, glycine can prevent excessive hydrogen peroxide production induced by glutamate in brain mitochondria [65], thereby reducing the prooxidant effects of the excessive glutamate concentrations.

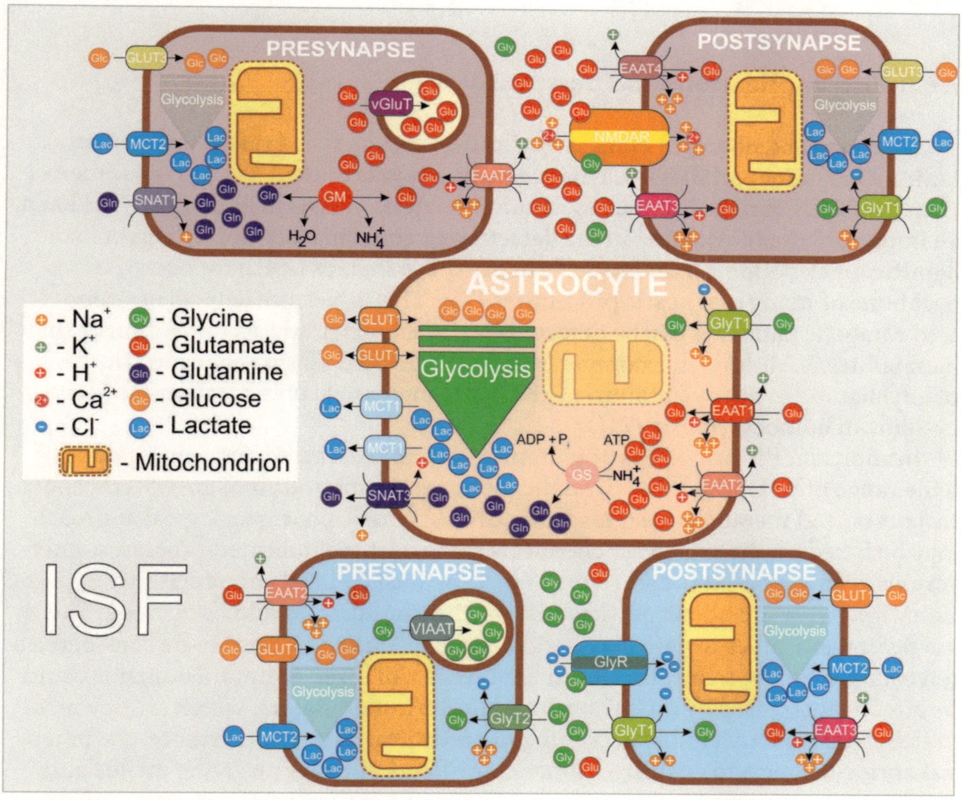

Figure 4.
The transport and activation of receptors in glycinergic and glutamatergic synapses. The transport system is tightly linked with glucose consumption. This transport system occurs in both astrocytes and neurons, but according to the ANLS model, the majority of glucose is consumed in astrocytes, with further diffusion of lactate to neurons. Lactate transport is facilitated by monocarboxylate transporters (MCTs), which have two different isoenzymes. MCT1 is expressed in astrocytes, and MCT2 is found in neurons [69]. Glutamate-glutamine cycling occurs between central astrocytes and neurons, mediated by sodium-coupled neutral amino acid transporters (SNATs). Transport is mediated by two isoforms, SNAT3 and SNAT1 [70]. ISF: interstitial fluid.

Interestingly, the effects of amino acids can vary depending on the species. For example, in a chick model, injections of L-glutamate, NMDA, and AMPA attenuated total distress vocalizations and induced sedation [66]. The association between glutamate and inhibition/sedation is even stronger because the brain contains a considerable level of glutamate decarboxylase, which directly catalyzes the decarboxylation of glutamate to GABA [27]. Additionally, glycine is not always associated with direct inhibition in the CNS. Indeed, in mature neurons, where there is a low intracellular Cl^- concentration maintained by K^+- Cl^- cotransporter 2 (KCC2), activation of GlyRs elicits an influx of Cl^-, leading to rapid hyperpolarization and postsynaptic inhibition [67]. In contrast, in immature neurons, activation of GlyRs results in efflux of Cl^-, leading to neuronal depolarization; this opens voltage-dependent Ca^{2+} channels, elicits action potentials, and establishes early network activity and excitation in the developing nervous system [68].

Thus, the balance between excitation and inhibition is the result of continuous interactions among different processes involving both glutamate and glycine. It is essential that the main reactions and regulatory sites are nonhomogenously distributed in neuronal space and are time-regulated. Convective flow does not restore the homogeneity of mediator and metabolite concentrations because of the tortuosity of the system [63]. A scheme of the balanced interactions between glycinergic and glutamatergic synapses is shown in **Figure 4**.

7. Clinical applications and perspectives

The first (and obvious) clinical application of AAs is as a reference level to indicate different pathologies. This suggestion covers more AAs than those mentioned above. For decades, the biochemical analysis of AAs in body fluids has been an important diagnostic tool in the detection of congenital errors of metabolism. Significant elevations of amino acids in plasma, urine, or CSF have been the backbone of many diagnostic procedures [71]. This is because defects in amino acid catabolic pathways can be detected by the characteristic accumulation of their metabolites. Well-known examples of this are elevated plasma concentrations of phenylalanine in phenylketonuria (PKU) and increased concentrations of homocysteine in homocystinuria [71].

In addition, the properties of glutamate/glycine discussed above indicate a wide range of potential medical applications for compounds that govern transport, receptors, and metabolic systems in the CNS. A classic pharmacological approach may be based on the search for chemicals that affect the indicated processes; interactions with the target protein site or reaction must be local and precisely unidirectional and wide metabolic participation of the candidate should be avoided. There are several examples to date. Each of the three mGlu subgroups can be considered a novel target for the treatment of schizophrenia. All three symptom domains could be effectively treated by mGlu5 positive allosteric modulators, which are devoid of toxicity and seizure liability according to preclinical data. Furthermore, the potential antipsychotic and cognitive-enhancing effects of drugs targeting mGlu1 and mGlu3 were supported by recent genetic investigations of schizophrenia patients [72]. Preclinical studies have revealed that specific mGluR subtypes mediate significant neuroprotective effects that reduce toxin-induced midbrain dopaminergic neuronal death in animal models of Parkinson's disease [41]. Additionally, mGluRs have emerged as research targets in treating Alzheimer's disease. In particular, mGluR-based compounds producing both symptomatic and disease-modifying effects in preclinical models of the disease are of special interest [73]. G protein-coupled mGluRs expressed by tumor cells, particularly cancer stem cells, might represent new candidate drug targets for the treatment of malignant brain tumors [74]. Group III mGluR agonists have been recently identified as promising tools for managing affective symptoms, such as the pathological anxiety observed in neuropathic pain. However, the use of mGluR ligands as anxiolytics was disappointing in clinical trials. Nevertheless, there is ground for a certain amount of optimism [75].

Pharmacological modulation of glycinergic inhibition could represent a novel therapeutic strategy for a variety of diseases involving altered synaptic inhibition, primarily in the spinal cord and brain stem but possibly also at supraspinal sites [74]. Among the inhibitors of GlyT-1, two candidates have attracted the most attention. Sarcosine, a known intermediate of glycine metabolism, had positive results as a short-term treatment of major depression and for acutely ill and chronically stable schizophrenia patients. Another GlyT-1 inhibitor, bitopertin, was expected to be effective in treating negative or positive schizophrenia symptoms. However, the phase III clinical trials fell short of the primary endpoint, and the investigation was halted due to its lack of efficacy in improving negative symptoms [76]. Gelsemium, a small genus of flowering plants from the family Loganiaceae, may be used as a pain treatment and for its mechanism of action. Gelsemium and its active alkaloids may produce antinociception by activating the spinal α3 glycine/allopregnanolone pathway in inflammatory, neuropathic, and bone cancer pain without inducing antinociceptive tolerance, in contrast to morphine [75].

Another strategy is to directly use AAs for medical treatment. In this scenario, glycine is the most appropriate candidate. Glycine has a wide spectrum of protective properties against different diseases and injuries. As such, it represents a novel anti-inflammatory, immunomodulatory and cytoprotective agent [77]. Oral supplementation of glycine at a proper dose is very successful in treating several metabolic disorders in individuals with cardiovascular diseases, various inflammatory diseases, cancers, diabetes, and obesity [34]. Glycine was well tolerated at a dose of 0.8 g/kg body weight a day, resulting in significantly increased serum glycine levels and a 7% reduction in negative symptoms in patients with treatment-resistant schizophrenia [78]. An acute high dosage of glycine attenuates the neurophysiological representation of the brain's preattentive acoustic change detection system (mismatch negativity) in healthy controls, raising the possibility that the optimal effects of glycine and other glycine agonists may depend on the integrity of the NMDA receptor system [79]. The glycine was effective in the treatment of ischaemic stroke patients. In a randomized, double-blind, placebo-controlled study on 200 patients with acute (<6 h) ischaemic stroke in the carotid artery area, 1.0–2.0 g/day of glycine was accompanied by a tendency towards decreased 30-day mortality (5.9% in the 1.0 g/day glycine and 10% in the 2.0 g/day glycine groups vs. 14% in the placebo and 14.3% in the 0.5 g/day glycine groups), an improved clinical outcome on the Orgogozo Stroke Scale ($p < 0.01$) and the Scandinavian Stroke Scale ($p < 0.01$) and a favorable functional outcome on the Barthel Index for Activities of Daily Living ($p < 0.01$) in the 1.0 g/day glycine group compared to those in the placebo group in patients with no or mild disability [80]. The molecular mechanism of such an effect is based on the ability of glycine to initiate stable vasodilatation of arterioles, which has been demonstrated in rat pial vessels and in mesenteric arterioles [81, 82].

8. Conclusions

According to experimental and clinical evidence, AAs are especially useful nutrients for the treatment of patients with different diseases. These nutrients not only supply a background pool for biochemical reactions, but the functions of the metabolites cover a wide range of neurochemical processes, and they are always

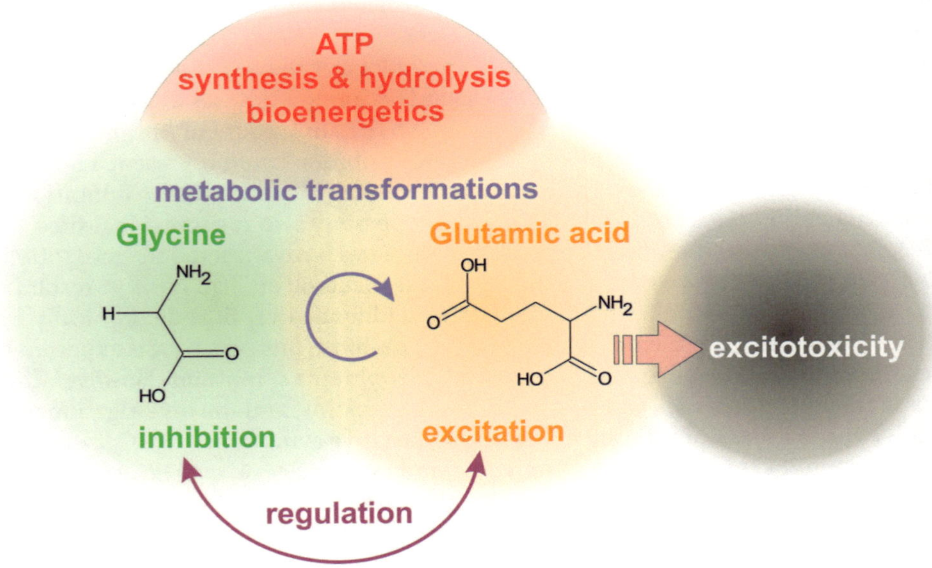

Figure 5.
Scheme of the mutual influence of inhibition and excitation mediated by glycine and glutamate.

mutually dependent. Even though some processes are decreased or increased in illnesses, it does not mean that the treatment strategy must be targeted to only correct the single altered process. A prominent example is glutamate-induced excitotoxicity in neurons. The best strategy to prevent increased glutamate concentrations is to maintain bioenergetic processes in neurons and astrocytes at high activity levels and to activate glycine-dependent processes. Moreover, it helps to assign the exceeded content of the neuromediator to a physiological range and to form stable conditions for further health development, avoiding excitotoxicity (**Figure 5**). Searching for exogenous antagonists of metabolic receptors seems to be an incorrect therapeutic strategy because the function of the AA-dependent system depends on the basic metabolic regulatory core of metabolic processes. Indeed, to find appropriate therapeutic methods, further fundamental and clinical investigations are necessary.

Conflict of interest

The author has no conflict of interest to declare.

Author details

Yaroslav R. Nartsissov
Institute of Cytochemistry and Molecular Pharmacology, Moscow, Russia

*Address all correspondence to: yarosl@biotic.dol.ru

References

[1] Parpura V, Verkhratsky A. Astroglial amino acid-based transmitter receptors. Amino Acids. 2013;**44**(4):1151-1158

[2] Magistretti PJ, Allaman I. A cellular perspective on brain energy metabolism and functional imaging. Neuron. 2015;**86**(4):883-901

[3] Blachier F, Mariotti F, Huneau JF, Tomé D. Effects of amino acid-derived luminal metabolites on the colonic epithelium and physiopathological consequences. Amino Acids. 2007;**33**(4):547-562

[4] Knights KM, Sykes MJ, Miners JO. Amino acid conjugation: Contribution to the metabolism and toxicity of xenobiotic carboxylic acids. Expert Opinion on Drug Metabolism and Toxicology. 2007;**3**(2):159-168

[5] Wu G. Amino acids: Metabolism, functions, and nutrition. Amino Acids. 2009;**37**(1):1-17

[6] Melendes-Hevia E, De Paz-lugo P, Cornish-Bowden A, Luz Cardenas M. A weak link in metabolism: the metabolic capacity for glycine biosynthesis does not satisfy the need for collagen synthesis. Journal Bioscience. 2009;**34**(6):853-872

[7] Wu G. Functional amino acids in growth, reproduction, and health. Advances in Nutrition. 2010;**1**(1):31-37

[8] DeFeudis FV. Amino acids as central neurotransmitters. Annual Review of Pharmacology. 1975;**15**:105-130

[9] Usherwood PN. Amino acids as neurotransmitters. Advances in Comparative Physiology and Biochemistry. 1978;**7**:227-309

[10] Avoli M, Krnjević K. The long and winding road to gamma-amino-butyric acid as neurotransmitter. Canadian Journal of Neurological Sciences. 2015;**43**(2):219-226

[11] Schousboe A, Apreza CL, Pasantes-Morales H. Gaba and taurine serve as respectively a neurotransmitter and an osmolyte in cultured cerebral cortical neurons. Advances in Experimental Medicine and Biology. 1992;**315**:391-397

[12] Morales HP, Schousboe A. Volume regulation in astrocytes: A role for taurine as an osmoeffector. Journal of Neuroscience Research. 1988;**20**(4): 505-509

[13] Hayashi MK. Structure-function relationship of transporters in the glutamate–glutamine cycle of the central nervous system. International Journal of Molecular Sciences. 2018;**19**(4):1-18

[14] Choi C, Ganji SK, Deberardinis RJ, Dimitrov IE, Pascual JM, Bachoo R, et al. Measurement of glycine in the human brain in vivo by 1H-MRS at 3 T: Application in brain tumors. Magnetic Resonance in Medicine. 2011;**66**(3): 609-618

[15] D'Souza DC, Gil R, Cassello K, Morrissey K, Abi-Saab D, White J, et al. IV glycine and oral D-cycloserine effects on plasma and CSF amino acids in healthy humans. Biological Psychiatry. 2000;**47**(5):450-462

[16] Beyoglu D, Idle JR. The glycine deportation system and its pharmacological consequences. Pharmacology and Therapeutics. 2012;**135**(2):151-167

[17] Zhou Y, Danbolt NC. Glutamate as a neurotransmitter in the healthy brain. Journal of Neural Transmission. 2014;**121**(8):799-817

[18] Juge N, Muroyama A, Hiasa M, Omote H, Moriyama Y. Vesicular inhibitory amino acid transporter is a

Cl-/ γ-aminobutyrate co-transporter. Journal of Biological Chemistry. 2009;**284**(50):35073-35078

[19] Hubbard JA, Binder DK. Chapter 9—Glutamate Metabolism. San Diego: Academic Press; 2016. pp. 197-224

[20] Duffield M, Patel A, Mortensen OV, Schnur D, Gonzalez-Suarez AD, Torres-Salazar D, et al. Transport rate of EAAT2 is regulated by amino acid located at the interface between the scaffolding and substrate transport domains. Neurochemistry International. 2020;**139**:1-13

[21] Harvey RJ, Yee BK. Glycine transporters as novel therapeutic targets in schizophrenia, alcohol dependence and pain. Nature Reviews Drug Discovery. 2013;**12**(11):866-885

[22] Grewer C, Gameiro A, Rauen T. SLC1 glutamate transporters. Pflugers Archiv European Journal of Physiology. 2014;**466**(1):3-24

[23] Kanai Y, Clémençon B, Simonin A, Leuenberger M, Lochner M, Weisstanner M, et al. The SLC1 high-affinity glutamate and neutral amino acid transporter family. Molecular Aspects of Medicine. 2013;**34**(2-3):108-120

[24] Dwyer D. Glucose metabolism in the brain. International Review of Neurobiology. 2002;**51**:1-535

[25] Pellerin L, Magistretti PJ. Sweet sixteen for ANLS. Journal of Cerebral Blood Flow and Metabolism. 2012;**32**(7):1152-1166

[26] Ashrafi G, Ryan TA. Glucose metabolism in nerve terminals. Current Opinion in Neurobiology. 2017;**45**:156-161

[27] Cooper AJL, Jeitner TM. Central role of glutamate metabolism in the maintenance of nitrogen homeostasis in normal and hyperammonemic brain. Biomolecules. 2016;**6**(2):1-33

[28] Eid T, Tu N, Lee T-SW, Lai JCK. Regulation of astrocyte glutamine synthetase in epilepsy. Neurochemistry International. 2013;**63**(7):670-681

[29] Massucci FA, DiNuzzo M, Giove F, Maraviglia B, Castillo IP, Marinari E, et al. Energy metabolism and glutamate-glutamine cycle in the brain: A stoichiometric modeling perspective. BMC Systems Biology. 2013;**7**:1-14

[30] McKenna MC, Stridh MH, McNair LF, Sonnewald U, Waagepetersen HS, Schousboe A. Glutamate oxidation in astrocytes: Roles of glutamate dehydrogenase and aminotransferases. Journal of Neuroscience Research. 2016;**94**(12):1561-1571

[31] Hong Y, Ren J, Zhang X, Wang W, Zeng AP. Quantitative analysis of glycine related metabolic pathways for one-carbon synthetic biology. Current Opinion in Biotechnology. 2020;**64**:70-78

[32] Kikuchi G, Motokawa Y, Yoshida T, Hiraga K. Glycine cleavage system: Reaction mechanism, physiological significance, and hyperglycinemia. Proceedings of the Japan Academy Series B: Physical and Biological Sciences. 2008;**84**(7):246-263

[33] Traynelis SF, Wollmuth LP, McBain CJ, Menniti FS, Vance KM, Ogden KK, et al. Glutamate receptor ion channels: Structure, regulation, and function. Pharmacological Reviews. 2010;**62**(3):405-496

[34] Razak MA, Begum PS, Viswanath B, Rajagopal S. Multifarious beneficial effect of nonessential amino acid, glycine: A review. Oxidative Medicine and Cellular Longevity. 2017;**2017**:1-8

[35] Paoletti P, Bellone C, Zhou Q. NMDA receptor subunit diversity: Impact on receptor properties, synaptic plasticity and disease. Nature Reviews Neuroscience. 2013;**14**(6):383-400

[36] Twomey EC, Sobolevsky AI. Structural mechanisms of gating in ionotropic glutamate receptors. Biochemistry. 2018;**57**(3):267-276

[37] Perez-Torres I, Zuniga-Munoz AM, Guarner-Lans V. Beneficial effects of the amino acid glycine. Mini Reviews in Medicinal Chemistry. 2017;**17**(1):15-32

[38] Petrat F, Boengler K, Schulz R, De Groot H. Glycine, a simple physiological compound protecting by yet puzzling mechanism(s) against ischaemia-reperfusion injury: current knowledge. British Journal of Pharmacology. 2012;**165**(7):2059-2072

[39] Ribeiro FM, Vieira LB, Pires RGW, Olmo RP, Ferguson SSG. Metabotropic glutamate receptors and neurodegenerative diseases. Pharmacological Research. 2017;**115**: 179-191

[40] Niswender CM, Conn PJ. Metabotropic glutamate receptors: Physiology, pharmacology, and disease. Annual Review of Pharmacology and Toxicology. 2010;**50**:295-322

[41] Masilamoni GJ, Smith Y. Metabotropic glutamate receptors: targets for neuroprotective therapies in Parkinson disease. Current Opinion in Pharmacology. 2018;**38**:72-80

[42] Ngomba RT, van Luijtelaar G. Metabotropic glutamate receptors as drug targets for the treatment of absence epilepsy. Current Opinion in Pharmacology. 2018;**38**:43-50

[43] Spampinato SF, Copani A, Nicoletti F, Sortino MA, Caraci F. Metabotropic glutamate receptors in glial cells: A new potential target for neuroprotection? Frontiers in Molecular Neuroscience. 2018;**11**:1-13

[44] Kumar A, Basak S, Rao S, Gicheru Y, Mayer ML, Sansom MSP, et al. Mechanisms of activation and desensitization of full-length glycine receptor in lipid nanodiscs. Nature. Communications. 2020;**11**(1):1-14

[45] Herguedas B, García-Nafría J, Cais O, Fernández-Leiro R, Krieger J, Ho H, et al. Structure and organization of heteromeric AMPA-type glutamate receptors. Science. 2016;**352**(6285):1-16

[46] Kumari J, Bendre AD, Bhosale S, Vinnakota R, Burada AP, Tria G, et al. Structural dynamics of the GluK3-kainate receptor neurotransmitter binding domains revealed by cryo-EM. International Journal of Biological Macromolecules. 2020;**149**:1051-1058

[47] Wang H, Lv S, Stroebel D, Zhang J, Pan Y, Huang X, et al. Gating mechanism and a modulatory niche of human GluN1-GluN2A NMDA receptors. Neuron. 2021;**109**(15):2443-2456

[48] Adeva-Andany M, Souto-Adeva G, Ameneiros-Rodríguez E, Fernández-Fernández C, Donapetry-García C, Domínguez-Montero A. Insulin resistance and glycine metabolism in humans. Amino Acids. 2018;**50**(1): 11-27

[49] Alvarado-Vasquez N, Lascurain R, Ceron E, Vanda B, Carvajal-Sandoval G, Tapia A, et al. Oral glycine administration attenuates diabetic complications in streptozotocin-induced diabetic rats. Life Sciences. 2006;**79**(3):225-232

[50] Koopman R, Caldow MK, Ham DJ, Lynch GS. Glycine metabolism in skeletal muscle: Implications for metabolic homeostasis. Current Opinion in Clinical Nutrition and Metabolic Care. 2017;**20**(4):237-242

[51] Van den Eynden J, Ali SS, Horwood N, Carmans S, Brone B, Hellings N, et al. Glycine and glycine receptor signalling in non-neuronal cells. Frontiers in Molecular Neuroscience. 2009;**2**(Aug):1-12

[52] Weinberg JM, Bienholz A, Venkatachalam MA. The role of glycine in regulated cell death. Cellular and Molecular Life Sciences. 2016;**73**(11-12): 2285-2308

[53] Choi DW. Excitotoxicity: Still hammering the ischemic brain in 2020. Frontiers in Neuroscience. 2020;**14**:1-27

[54] Fern R, Matute C. Glutamate receptors and white matter stroke. Neuroscience Letters. 2019;**694**:86-92

[55] Szydlowska K, Tymianski M. Calcium, ischemia and excitotoxicity. Cell Calcium. 2010;**47**(2):122-129

[56] Featherstone DE, Shippy SA. Regulation of synaptic transmission by ambient extracellular glutamate. Neuroscientist. 2008;**14**(2):171-181

[57] Olloquequi J, Cornejo-Córdova E, Verdaguer E, Soriano FX, Binvignat O, Auladell C, et al. Excitotoxicity in the pathogenesis of neurological and psychiatric disorders: Therapeutic implications. Journal of Psychopharmacology. 2018;**32**(3):265-275

[58] Esposito Z, Belli L, Toniolo S, Sancesario G, Bianconi C, Martorana A. Amyloid β, glutamate, excitotoxicity in alzheimer's disease: Are we on the right track? CNS Neuroscience and Therapeutics. 2013;**19**(8):549-555

[59] Iovino L, Tremblay ME, Civiero L. Glutamate-induced excitotoxicity in Parkinson's disease: The role of glial cells. Journal of Pharmacological Sciences. 2020;**144**(3):151-164

[60] Sepers MD, Raymond LA. Mechanisms of synaptic dysfunction and excitotoxicity in Huntington's disease. Drug Discovery Today. 2014;**19**(7):990-996

[61] Mehta A, Prabhakar M, Kumar P, Deshmukh R, Sharma PL. Excitotoxicity: Bridge to various triggers in neurodegenerative disorders. European Journal of Pharmacology. 2013;**698**(1-3):6-18

[62] Chiu DN, Jahr CE. Extracellular glutamate in the nucleus accumbens is nanomolar in both synaptic and non-synaptic compartments. Cell Reports. 2017;**18**(11):2576-2583

[63] Selivanov VA, Zagubnaya OA, Nartsissov YR, Cascante M. Unveiling a key role of oxaloacetate-glutamate interaction in regulation of respiration and ROS generation in nonsynaptic brain mitochondria using a kinetic model. PLoS ONE. 2021;**16**(8):e0255164

[64] Selin AA, Lobysheva NV, Nesterov SV, Skorobogatova YA, Byvshev IM, Pavlik LL, et al. On the regulative role of the glutamate receptor in mitochondria. Biological Chemistry. 2016;**397**(5):445-458

[65] Lobysheva NV, Selin AA, Vangeli IM, Byvshev IM, Yaguzhinsky LS, Nartsissov YR. Glutamate induces H2O2 synthesis in nonsynaptic brain mitochondria. Free Radical Biology and Medicine. 2013;**65**:428-435

[66] Furuse M. Screening of central functions of amino acids and their metabolites for sedative and hypnotic effects using chick models. European Journal of Pharmacology. 2015;**762**: 382-393

[67] Benarroch EE. Glycine and its synaptic interactions: Functional and clinical implications. Neurology. 2011;**77**(7):677-683

[68] Doyon N, Vinay L, Prescott SA, De Koninck Y. Chloride regulation: A dynamic equilibrium crucial for synaptic inhibition. Neuron. 2016;**89**(6):1157-1172

[69] Weiler A, Volkenhoff A, Hertenstein H, Schirmeier S. Metabolite transport across the mammalian and

insect brain diffusion barriers. Neurobiology of Disease. 2017;**107**:15-31

[70] Mackenzie B, Erickson JD. Sodium-coupled neutral amino acid (System N/A) transporters of the SLC38 gene family. Pflugers Archiv European Journal of Physiology. 2004;**447**(5): 784-795

[71] de Koning TJ. Amino acid synthesis deficiencies. Journal of Inherited Metabolic Disease. 2017;**40**(4):609-620

[72] Stansley BJ, Conn PJ. The therapeutic potential of metabotropic glutamate receptor modulation for schizophrenia. Current Opinion in Pharmacology. 2018;**38**:31-36

[73] Caraci F, Nicoletti F, Copani A. Metabotropic glutamate receptors: the potential for therapeutic applications in Alzheimer's disease. Current Opinion in Pharmacology. 2018;**38**:1-7

[74] Iacovelli L, Orlando R, Rossi A, Spinsanti P, Melchiorri D, Nicoletti F. Targeting metabotropic glutamate receptors in the treatment of primary brain tumors. Current Opinion in Pharmacology. 2018;**38**:59-64

[75] Ferraguti F. Metabotropic glutamate receptors as targets for novel anxiolytics. Current Opinion in Pharmacology. 2018;**38**:37-42

[76] Yao L, Zhou Q. Enhancing NMDA receptor function: Recent progress on allosteric modulators. Neural Plasticity. 2017;**2017**:1-11

[77] Zhong Z, Wheeler MD, Li X, Froh M, Schemmer P, Yin M, et al. L-glycine: A novel antiinflammatory, immunomodulatory, and cytoprotective agent. Current Opinion in Clinical Nutrition and Metabolic Care. 2003;**6**(2):229-240

[78] Heresco-Levy U, Javitt DC, Ermilov M, Mordel C, Horowitz A, Kelly D. Double-blind, placebo-controlled, crossover trial of glycine adjuvant therapy for treatment-resistant schizophrenia. British Journal of Psychiatry. 1996;**169**(5):610-617

[79] Leung S, Croft RJ, O'Neill BV, Nathan PJ. Acute high-dose glycine attenuates mismatch negativity (MMN) in healthy human controls. Psychopharmacology. 2008;**196**(3): 451-460

[80] Gusev EI, Skvortsova VI, Dambinova SA, Raevskiy KS, Alekseev AA, Bashkatova VG, et al. Neuroprotective effects of glycine for therapy of acute ischaemic stroke. Cerebrovascular Diseases. 2000;**10**(1):49-60

[81] Podoprigora GI, Nartsissov YR, Aleksandrov PN. Effect of glycine on microcirculation in pial vessels of rat brain. Bulletin of Experimental Biology and Medicine. 2005;**139**(6):675-677

[82] Podoprigora GI, Nartsissov YR. Effect of glycine on the microcirculation in rat mesenteric vessels. Bulletin of Experimental Biology and Medicine. 2009;**147**(3):308-311

Chapter 6

Emerging Roles of Non-Coding RNA in Neuronal Function and Dysfunction

Steven G. Fagan and Shona Pfeiffer

Abstract

Advancements in RNA sequencing technologies in recent years have contributed greatly to our understanding of the transcriptome and the now widely recognized multifaceted functions of RNA. The discovery and functional analysis of an increasing number of novel small non-coding RNAs (ncRNAs) has highlighted their importance as critical regulators of gene expression and brain function. In particular, two diverse classes of ncRNAs, microRNAs (miRNAs) and tRNA-derived small RNAs (tsRNAs), are especially abundant in the nervous system and play roles in regulation of gene expression and protein translation, cellular stress responses and complex underlying pathophysiology of neurological diseases. This chapter will discuss the most recent findings highlighting the dysregulation, functions and regulatory roles of ncRNAs in the pathophysiological mechanisms of neurological disorders and their relevance as novel biomarkers of injury and therapeutic agents.

Keywords: non-coding RNA (ncRNA), microRNA (miRNA), tRNA-derived small RNAs (tsRNA), tRNA-derived stress-induced RNA (tiRNA), tRNA fragments (tRFs), epigenetics, molecular biology, neurological disorders

1. Introduction

Normal neuronal function and development is reliant on tightly controlled regulation of gene expression at many levels. Advancements in transcriptomics and functional validation has elucidated key biological roles for non-coding RNAs (ncRNAs), transcripts do not encode proteins, in the regulation of a wide range of neuronal functions and pathophysiological processes. Over the past two decades large international collaborative research efforts such as the Human Genome Project and the ENCODE (Encyclopedia of DNA Elements) project have estimated that approximately 80% of the mammalian genome transcribes ncRNA and that 97% of RNA transcripts in the cell are non-coding [1–3]. This remarkable and unexplored area of molecular biology has since yielded many more types of ncRNA that have been shown to play a crucial role in a variety of biological processes.

ncRNA are classified either by their length or by functionality (**Table 1**). Small ncRNA are considered transcripts <200 nucleotides (nts) in length and long ncRNA are those >200 nts. Housekeeping ncRNA are constitutively expressed and are involved in mechanisms of cellular activity that are vital for cell viability. These include rRNA, tRNA and the more recently identified small nuclear RNA (snRNA), small nucleolar RNA (snoRNA) and telomerase RNA (TERC). Regulatory ncRNA

Class	Abbreviation	Full name	Size (nts)
Housekeeping RNAs	rRNA	Ribosomal RNA	120–4500
	snoRNA	Small nucleolar RNA	60–400
	snRNA	Small nuclear RNA	100–300
	tRNA	Transfer RNA	76–90
	TERC	Telomerase RNA	—
Regulatory RNAs	circRNA	Circular RNA	100–10,000
	eRNA	Enhancer RNA	50–2000
	lncRNA	Long non-coding RNA	>200
	tsRNA	tRNA-derived small RNA	16–50
	piRNA	piwi-interacting RNA	26–32
	siRNA	Small interfering RNA	20–25
	miRNA	microRNA	21–23
	Y RNA	—	—

Table 1.
Classification of ncRNAs.

regulate gene expression through epigenetic, transcriptional and post-transcriptional mechanisms, and include microRNA (miRNA), tRNA-derived small RNA (tsRNA), piwi-interacting RNA (piRNA), long non-coding RNA (lncRNA) and circular RNA (circRNA) [4].

This chapter will focus on two classes of ncRNA, miRNA and tsRNA, which are highly enriched in the central nervous system (CNS) with important roles in neuronal function and dysfunction. The central roles played by these classes of ncRNAs and their dysregulation in disease, particularly their ability to regulate multiple genes, place them as promising biomarkers and therapeutic targets, entering many clinical trials.

2. microRNA

2.1 miRNA biogenesis and mechanism of action

miRNAs are transcribed by RNA polymerase II/III from either independent miRNA genes (monocistronic), as clusters of up to a few hundred miRNA (polycistronic) or from the introns of protein-coding genes (intronic). Approximately half of miRNAs are considered intronic, however a functional relationship between miRNAs and host genes is rarely found. Long primary miRNA (pri-miRNA) transcripts are processed in the nucleus by a microprocessor complex containing ribonuclease III, Drosha, and RNA-binding protein subunit DGCR8 (DiGeorge syndrome critical region 8). Cleavage of the pri-miRNA by Drosha results in a 2 nt 3′ overhang and the characteristic 'hairpin' structure of the 65 nt precursor miRNA (pre-miRNA). The pre-miRNA is then exported to the cytosol by the exportin-5 (XPO5)/RanGTP complex, where it is further processed by the endonuclease Dicer, removing the terminal loop resulting in a double stranded miRNA containing the mature miRNA guide strand and passenger strand, typically 21 – 23 nts in length (**Figure 1A**).

The RNA-induced silencing complex (RISC) is a heterogeneous multi-protein complex that uses one miRNA strand as a template to target complimentary mRNAs

DOI: http://dx.doi.org/10.5772/intechopen.101327

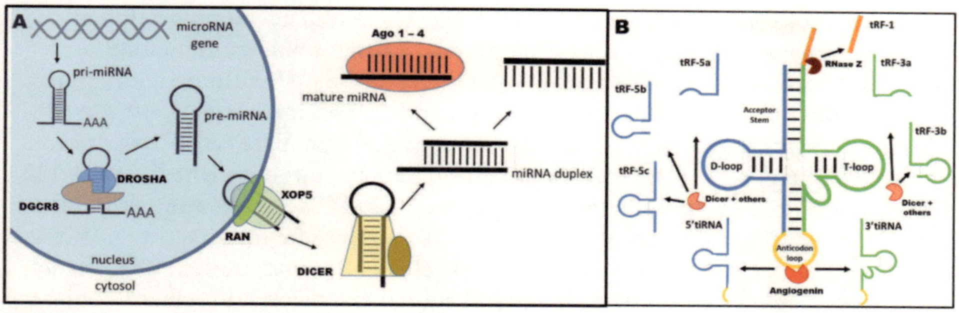

Figure 1.
Illustration of the biogenesis of (A) miRNA and (B) tsRNA.

for degradation or translational repression, post-transcriptionally regulating gene expression. The double-stranded miRNA duplex is loaded into a binding pocket within an Argonaute family (Ago1-4) protein, which constitutes the principal component of RISC, mediated by Hsc70/Hsp90. The miRNA is unwound to single-stranded miRNAs and one 'guide strand' is anchored into the Ago protein, determining the specificity of the RISC, while the passenger strand is subject to degradation. The directionality of the mature miRNA guide strand originating from the 5′ or 3′ arm of the pre-miRNA duplex determines the miRNA-5p and -3p species. While typically one strand is preferentially loaded, for some miRNA duplexes both arms can give rise to functional mature miRNAs that can be loaded into Ago proteins and used to guide the RISC to mRNA transcripts.

Recognition of target mRNA occurs by complementary base pairing between the miRNA seed region (2–8 nt) of the 5′ end of the guide strand and the mRNA transcript, typically within the 3′ UTR; however miRNA can also bind within mRNA promoter regions, the coding sequence, and 5′ UTR. The Ago protein present and the degree of complementarity between the guide and target strand determines the mechanism of gene silencing, triggering target degradation or translational repression. Importantly, the short seed sequence requirement for mRNA targeting confers ability for individual miRNAs to target multiple genes across several different pathways. Similarly, an individual mRNA may contain target sites for multiple miRNAs, placing miRNAs in a powerful position in the regulation and modulation of the transcriptomic landscape. Dysregulation of miRNAs, therefore, has significant implications and consequences for biological functions in physiological and pathological conditions.

2.2 miRNA functions

2.2.1 Neuronal development and function

An extensive catalog of work has demonstrated the involvement of miRNAs across the development, function and maintenance of the CNS. The cell-specific deletion of Dicer inhibits the maturation of miRNA and has been shown to delay embryonic CNS development, alter dendritic and spine morphology and lead to early postnatal death [5–7]. Specific miRNAs have been identified with central roles in regulation of adult neural stem cell proliferation [8–10] and the differentiation of cells into specific neuronal sub-types [11–14]. Post-transcriptional regulation of N-cadherin expression by the miR-379-410 cluster mediates neuronal migration [15] and miR-132 is involved in the activity-dependent integration of neurons into the adult dentate gyrus [16].

The controlled extension of neuronal processes as well as the generation of adaptable synapses are key in the development of functional neural networks in the CNS. A number of miRNAs have been closely associated with the regulation of axonal and dendritic morphology, and synaptic plasticity. Neurite outgrowth is highly dependent on extracellular trophic cues that stimulate cAMP response element binding protein (CREB) transcription factor, a target of which is miR-132. In axons, miR-132 downregulates the activity of the GTPase-activating protein p250 GAP resulting in axonal sprouting [17]. A number of counteracting miRNAs tightly regulate axonal length. The miR-17/92 cluster downregulates *PTEN* resulting in activation of the mTOR pathway and axonal extension [18], whereas miR-9 has been shown to locally repress *Map1b* expression and inhibit axonal growth [19]. Conversely, miR-9 promotes dendritic development and its loss results in reduced dendritic length and complexity [20]. Similar to axonal extension, miR-132 has been shown to positively regulate dendritic length, arborization and spine density in dendritic extensions in an activity-dependent manner [21, 22]. miR-132-mediated regulation of spine density has been attributed to its direct association with matrix metalloproteinase-9 [23] and miR-132-medited repression of p250GAP in dendritic spines has been associated with Leptin-induced synaptogenesis [24]. In *Drosophila melanogaster* miR-284 has been shown to affect the expression of the glutamate receptors GluRIIA and GluRIIB indicating a role in the regulation of synaptic strength [25] and in higher order animals the inhibition of miR-132 and miR-219 have been associated with disturbed circadian rhythm and the impairment of memory acquisition [26].

2.2.2 Inflammation

Inflammation in the CNS is an important process for the alleviation of infection or the resolution of cerebral damage; however, aberrant or chronic inflammation has been implicated in a number of neurological disorders [27]. Microglial cells, the resident immune cells of the CNS, are enriched in a number of miRNAs [28] and expression of these is altered in response to inflammatory stimuli [29]. Specific miRNAs have been associated with the development of a pro- or anti-inflammatory phenotype. miR-155 is a well-studied pro-inflammatory mediator in macrophages and microglia, targeting a number of anti-inflammatory regulators for degradation induced in response to NF-κB dependent TLR signaling. Furthermore, p53-mediated induction of miR-155 is known to target anti-inflammatory transcription factor *c-Maf*, resulting in a pro-inflammatory reaction [30]. miR-124 and miR-146a are both widely reported negative regulators of CNS inflammation, down-regulating inflammatory mediators. miR-146a is also induced through TLR/NF-κB-dependent signaling in response to various immune mediators, and subsequently reduces NF-κB transcriptional activity. miR-146a expression is inversely correlated with inflammatory-related proteins [31]. Similarly miR-124, a highly abundant neuronal and immune cell miRNA, has been reported to negatively regulate TLR signaling [32] promote microglial quiescence, and reduce microglial MHC-II, TNF-α and ROS production [33].

2.2.3 Apoptosis

Neuronal cell death is a key feature in neurodegenerative diseases and has been shown to involve a number of miRNAs. In models of spinal cord injury, activation of miR-21-5p and miR-494 as well as the inhibition of miR-29b, reduced apoptosis through stimulation of the AKT/mTOR signaling pathway [34–36]. Specific miRNAs have been shown to have a more direct effect on the apoptotic cascade. Indeed, the inhibition of miR-24, miR-497, miR-15a/16-1, miR-181a and miR-106b-5p increases expression of anti-apoptotic proteins Bcl-w, Bcl-2 and Bcl-xl resulting in attenuation of neuronal apoptosis [37–41].

3. tsRNA

Previously thought of as simple degradation products, tsRNA are cleaved fragments of full tRNA transcripts. In eukaryotes, tRNA genes are transcribed by polymerase III and the 5′ leader sequence and 3′ trailer sequences are removed from the pre-tRNA sequence by the endonucleases RNase P and RNase Z, respectively [42–44]. The mature tRNA is generated by the addition of a CCA tail by CCase [45, 46]. Mature tRNAs are 73–90 nt long with a classic 'cloverleaf' secondary structure consisting of an anti-codon loop that recognizes mRNA codons, an acceptor stem that binds amino acids, a dihydrouridine (D) loop, a thymidine (T) loop and a variable (V) loop [47]. tRNA are a highly modified species with over 170 independent modifications reported to date [48]. These modifications are largely localized on the anticodon loop, affecting the speed and accuracy of decoding, or the structural core of the molecule affecting stability and degradation pathways [49, 50]. tsRNA are generated from the cleavage of tRNA by endonucleases and are classified by their cleavage site and length as either tRNA-derived stress-induced RNA (tiRNA) or tRNA fragments (tRFs).

3.1 Biogenesis and structure of tsRNA

3.1.1 tiRNA

The generation of tiRNA occurs when the stress-induced RNase angiogenin (Ang) cleaves mature tRNA at the anticodon loop [51]. This produces transcripts 31–40 nts long that are defined as either 5′ or 3′tiRNA depending of the presence of a 3′ or 5′ end at the anticodon loop respectively (**Figure 1B**). The production of Ang is mediated by the transcription factor hypoxia-inducible factor-1α (HIF-1α) and thus tiRNA generation is closely linked with cellular stress [52]. Accumulation of tiRNA is known to occur following oxidative stress, heat shock, UV radiation, hypoxia and starvation [53–56].

3.1.2 tRF

tRFs are shorter transcripts of 14–30 nts that are produced by cleavage of tRNA at the D-loop, T-loop or stem region by Ang, Dicer and another yet to be identified member of the RNase superfamily [57]. Cleavage of tRNA at the D-loop generates fragments of three different lengths—tRF-5a (14–16 nts), tRF-5b (22–24 nts) or tRF-5c (28–30 nts). Similarly, cleavage at the T-loop produces tRF-3a (18 nt) or tRF-3b (22 nt). The cleavage of pre-tRNA at the 3′ end results in the generation of tRF-1 (**Figure 1B**) [57, 58].

3.2 tsRNA mechanism of action

3.2.1 Gene silencing

Similar to miRNAs, tRFs have been associated with the epigenetic regulator RISC, however mechanistic details on the role of tsRNA in the RISC remain to be elucidated. A recent meta-analysis of short RNA libraries from HEK293 cells demonstrated that both tRF-3 and tRF-5 associate with Ago proteins; however, a preference for Ago1, 3 and 4 over Ago2 was identified [59]. Interestingly a subsequent study in *D. melanogaster* revealed an age-related shift in tRF-Ago binding demonstrating a preference for Ago2 binding over Ago1 with increasing age [60].

3.2.2 Regulation of protein translation

The synthesis of protein is a central activity in all cells that consumes a high level of energy and is dynamic in response to metabolic conditions and external stimuli. The regulation of protein translation therefore is a vital process in the maintenance of cell viability and the stress response. Canonical cap-dependent translation begins with the formation of the eukaryotic initiation factor (eIF) 4F complex containing eIF4A, a DEAD-box helicase, eIF4E and eIF4G. The eIF4E subunit binds to the 5' m7GTP cap on target mRNA and the eIF4G subunit is a scaffold protein that mediates the recruitment of other proteins including eIF3 and poly(A) binding protein (PABP). eIF4F binding to the 5′ m7GTP cap and the 3′ poly(A) tail circularizes the target mRNA and allows the 48S pre-initiation complex, containing the 40S small ribosomal subunit, Met-$tRNA_i^{met}$ and eIF2, to scan the 5′ untranslated region and find the AUG start codon [61].

The dynamic regulation of protein translation in response to cellular stress and metabolic conditions is vital to cell survival. Stress-induced Ang-generated 5′tiRNA have been shown to halt the initiation of protein translation and facilitate the packaging of stalled translational complexes into stress granules [54]. Stress granules are cytoplasmic RNA-protein complexes that rapidly assemble and disassemble in response to cellular stress. This sequestration allows for the utilization of energy stores elsewhere and the recommencement of protein translation under optimum conditions [62]. Specific 5′tiRNA that contain a terminal oligoguanine (TOG) motif form stable G-quadruplex (G4) structures that directly bind the HEAT domain of eIF4G displacing eIF4A and inhibiting scanning of the mRNA target. Furthermore, 5′tiRNA with a 5′ monophosphate modification have been shown to bind the RNA binding protein YB-1 via the cold shock domain to precipitate the formation of stress granules [63].

Current knowledge on the effect of tRFs on protein translation is less advanced. Research in prokaryotic cells has demonstrated that tRF-5c of Val-GAC can bind the small ribosomal subunit and interfere with peptidyl transferase activity thereby inhibiting protein translation [64, 65]. In eukaryotic cells the tRF-3b of Gly-GCC reduced the level of specific protein with no concomitant reduction on mRNA levels indicating regulation at the translational level [66].

3.3 tsRNA functions

3.3.1 tsRNA and apoptosis

Disruption to the tsRNA system has been associated with increased cell death. Hypo-methylation of tRNA that arises from the inhibition of NSun2 increases cleavage by Ang and the accumulation of 5′tiRNA. The subsequent sustained depression in protein translation results in neuronal shrinkage, impaired synapse formation, cell death and is associated with neurodevelopmental deficiencies [67]. Loss-of-function mutations in the RNA kinase CLP1 has been shown to increase the level of tyrosine pre-tRNA fragments resulting in exaggerated p53 activation and vulnerability to cell death in cells exposed to oxidative stress [68]. Conversely, Ang has been shown to reduce cell death in neurons exposed to hyperosmotic stress in a tiRNA-mediated fashion. Specific Ang-generated tiRNA interact with cytochrome c and form a ribonucleoprotein complex that limits the formation of apoptosomes and reduces caspase-3 activation [53].

3.3.2 tsRNA and inflammation

Little research has been carried out on the involvement of tsRNA in the immune system; however, the expression of 5′tiRNA and tRF5 has been reported in mouse leukocytes and human monocytes respectively [69]. It is possible that tsRNAs play a regulatory role in the cellular response to inflammatory signals. In human chondrocytes, the pro-inflammatory cytokine IL-1β was shown to increase the expression of specific tRF-3s [70]. These fragments downregulated the cytokine signaling molecule JAK3 in an Ago-dependent manner. Furthermore, tsRNA may possess the ability to stimulate the immune response with reports demonstrating that tsRNA bind directly to Toll-like receptors on T-helper 1 and cytotoxic T cells [71].

4. ncRNA in neurological disease

4.1 Parkinson's disease

Parkinson's disease (PD) is characterized by the progressive loss of dopaminergic neurons resulting in the deterioration of motor function. Altered expression of miR-133b has been reported in the midbrain of PD patients. This is notable as the transcription factor *Pitx3* is a target of miR-133b and is involved in the maturation and function of dopaminergic neurons [12]. Gain-of-function mutations to the leucine-rich repeat kinase 2 (LRRK2) has been closely associated with both sporadic and inherited forms of PD [72]. A reduction in miR-205 has been observed in sporadic PD patients with increased LRRK2 protein expression. Furthermore, *in vitro* studies revealed that miR-205 reduces LRRK2 expression and alleviates its neurodegenerative effect [73]. Conversely, LRRK2 has been shown to disrupt miR-187* and let-7-mediated regulation of protein translation resulting in a pathogenic overproduction of E2F1/DP [74]. Another PD-related gene *SNCA* has been reported as a potential target of miR-7, miR-153 and miR-433 [75, 76]. miR-124 has been reported to play protective roles in dopaminergic neuronal apoptosis and autophagy in PD by regulating the AMPK/mTOR pathway. Suppression of miR-124 was been shown to regulate AMPK/mTOR signaling, significantly increasing p-AMPK activity and autophagy-associated Beclin 1 and LC3 II/LC3 I ratio [77].

In two independent studies, variations to the tsRNA-generating enzyme Ang have been reported in a subset of PD patients [78, 79]. Altered expression of tsRNA have also been reported in the amygdala [80], prefrontal cortex, cerebral spinal fluid and serum of PD patients [81]. Further work is required to elucidate the involvement of tsRNA in the pathogenesis of PD.

4.2 Alzheimer's disease

Alzheimer's disease (AD) is an age-related neurodegenerative disorder characterized by the progressive loss of cognition and memory due to severe neuronal cell loss. Hallmarks of the disease include the formation of extracellular amyloid plaques and intracellular neurofibrillary tangles of hyperphosphorylated tau. Given the high degree of cell death and chronic inflammation in the CNS, it is unsurprising that a large number of miRNAs are differentially expressed in AD [82–85], however, a number of miRNAs have also been shown to affect the pathogenic mechanisms of the disease.

Alternative splicing of amyloid precursor protein (APP), the parent molecule of pathogenic Aβ, is regulated by miR-124. Indeed, miR-124 is downregulated in the AD brain and its expression was shown to inhibit polypyrimidine tract binding protein 1 (PTBP1) resulting in increased APP with exon 7 and 8 inclusion [86]. Alterations of this kind have been associated with increased Aβ production [87]. Furthermore, miR-98 reduces the expression of insulin-like growth factor 1 (IGF-1) which is involved in the processing of APP. Overexpression of miR-98 downregulates IGF-1 resulting in increased Aβ production and tau phosphorylation [88]. The expression of tau is affected by the levels of miR-34a and miR-26b [89, 90]. Overexpression of miR-26b also leads to aberrant cell cycle entry that involves the nuclear export and activation of cyclin-dependent kinase 5 (CDK5), a major kinase involved in tau phosphorylation [89]. Finally, pro-inflammatory NFκB-associated miRNAs such as miR-7, miR-9, miR-34a, miR-125b, miR-46a and miR-155 are all upregulated in AD [85]. Presenilin 2 (PS2) mutations have been implicated in the development of autosomal dominant AD, and microglial knockout of PS2 reduces miR-146 expression and results in an increased pro-inflammatory response [91]. The level of inflammation in the CNS is a strong determining factor for disease progression in AD [92].

Limited work has been carried out to date on the involvement of tsRNA in AD; however, similar to PD, mutation of tsRNA-generating enzyme Ang has been identified. In an Italian cohort of AD patients nonsense mutations in *ANG* were identified with 0.2% frequency resulting in a 51 amino acid shortening in the protein [93].

4.3 Stroke

Stroke remains one of the leading causes of death and disability worldwide, conferring a high morbidity, disability, and mortality. Cerebral ischaemia triggers a complex cascade of physiological, biochemical and gene expression changes primarily resulting from impaired cellular energetics and the collapse of ion gradients. In particular, ischaemia-mediated glutamate elevation and subsequent over-activation of glutamate N-methyl-D-aspartate (NMDA) receptors is central to excitotoxic neuronal injury and cell death during ischaemic stroke [94, 95].

miR-107 has been shown to play a key role in the regulation of excitotoxicity in ischaemic neuronal injury, associated with increased glutamate accumulation both *in vivo* and in ischaemic stroke patients [96]. Increased miR-107 following ischaemic stroke inhibits GLT-1 expression, an abundant glutamate transporter, resulting in the accumulation of glutamate. Hypoxamir miR-210 has been widely reported as a miRNA ubiquitously expressed in ischaemic cells and tissues, with a central role in adaptation to low-oxygen environments such as tumourigenesis and ischaemia [97]. Robust induction of miR-210-3p following ischaemic stroke *in vivo* has been associated with modulation of PI3K-p70S6K signaling in response to AMPK activation and NMDA receptor-mediated glutamate excitotoxicity [98]. A number of other miRNAs have also been reported to play roles in the regulation of glutamate neurotransmission and excitotoxicity in ischaemic stroke, including miR-223, miR-181, miR-125a, miR-125b, miR-1000, miR-132 and miR-124a [99].

miR-223 has been shown to regulate the functional expression of glutamate receptor AMPAR subunit GluR2 and NMDAR subunit NR2B, which control neuronal excitability in response to glutamate, reducing neuronal excitability and cell death by inhibition of NMDA-induced calcium influx in hippocampal neurons [100]. One of the most abundantly expressed neuronal miRNAs, dysregulation of miR-124 has been implicated in many CNS disorders and has been shown to be downregulated following ischaemic stroke [101]. Downregulation of miR-124 *in vivo* following ischaemic stroke has been associated with upregulation of death-associated protein kinase 1 (DAPK1), identified as a direct target of miR-124, caspase-3, and cleaved caspase-3, while over-expression of miR-124 was shown to significantly decrease DAPK1, caspase-3, cleaved caspase-3 levels and reduce

NMDA- and oxygen-glucose deprivation (OGD)-induced neuronal death *in vivo* [102]. Moreover, the neuroprotective role of miR-124 has been associated with decreased expression of pro-apoptotic protein Bax and increased expression of anti-apoptotic Bcl-2 and Bcl-xl [103].

In the context of inflammation associated with cerebral ischaemia, miR-181c has been shown to inhibit prominent pro-inflammatory cytokine TNF-α in response to OGD, reducing microglial activation and neuronal cell death [104]. Furthermore, miR-216a, miR-3437b and miR-126-3p or -5p have also been associated with regulation of TNF following cerebral ischaemia.

Recent studies have shown tiRNAs to be upregulated following ischaemia in models of OGD *in vitro* and following ischaemic-reperfusion injury *in vivo.* Rapid and response-specific increases in tiRNA levels have been shown to correlate with degree of tissue damage, highlighting the potential role of tiRNA detection as a stress biomarker of injury [55, 56, 105, 106]. Furthermore, upregulation of 5′tiRNA fragments has been shown to inhibit endothelial angiogenesis following ischaemic stroke, indicating a role in modulating cerebral responses to ischaemic injury [106].

4.4 Amyolateral sclerosis

Amyolateral sclerosis (ALS) is the third most common neurodegenerative disease and is characterized by the rapid degeneration of cortical and spinal motor neurons leading to paralysis and death within 3–5 years of diagnosis [107, 108]. Approximately 90% of cases are sporadic, however a number of genetic mutations have been identified that account for 11% of sporadic and 70% of familial ALS [107, 109]. Mutations involving superoxide dismutase (SOD1), fused in sarcoma (FUS), TAR DNA-binding protein 43 (TDP43) and a hexanucleotide repeat expansion on chromosome 9 in open reading frame 72 (C9ORF72) have all been associated with ALS pathology [109].

Deregulation of miR-142-3p has been identified in both SOD1 and TDP-43 mutant mice, as well as in serum from ALS patients. Subsequent bioinformatic analysis identified TDP-43 and C9orf72 as targets of miR-142-3p, further implicating this miRNA in ALS pathology [110]. The skeletal muscle-specific miRNA, miR-206, regulates myogenesis, promotes the formation of neuromuscular junctions and is upregulated in ALS [111, 112]. This protective response occurs early in disease progression and plateaus [111], and higher levels of miR-206 are found in spinal ALS which is associated with lower atrophy rates [113]. Upregulation of miR-155 has been identified in both sporadic and familial ALS, and its inhibition in SOD1 mutant mice resulted in increased survival [114]. Finally, a number of miRNA associated with regulation of oxidative stress are altered in ALS. X-linked inhibitor of apoptosis (XIAP) and the Nrf2-ARE pathway have been closely associated with neuronal dysfunction in ALS and are regulated by miR-34a and miR-27a [115, 116].

As seen with other neurodegenerative diseases, mutations to *ANG* have been identified in ALS and repeatedly validated in independent cohorts [79, 117–119]. Characterization of these mutations determined a reduction in ribonuclease activity and nuclear translocation of Ang [117]. Interestingly, the Ang-generated tiRNA 5′ValCAC is increased in $SOD1^{G93A}$ mice at symptom onset and correlate with Ang expression and slower disease progression. Furthermore, increased 5′ValCAC in ALS patient serum samples is correlated with slower disease progression [120].

4.5 Epilepsy

Epilepsy is a heterogeneous group of disorders characterized by spontaneous and recurrent seizures that affects approximately 50 million people worldwide [121].

In the majority of instances, seizures can be controlled, however approximately 30% of cases are treatment resistant. Seizures arise from abnormal synchronous activity in hyperexcitable neuronal networks and while this can be attributed to altered electrophysiological properties of ion channels and neurotransmitter systems, converging lines of research have also indicated a central role for the regulation of protein translation [122, 123].

As described in Section 2.2.1, miRNAs play a key role in neuronal excitability and connectivity making them prime targets in epilepsy research. The growth, spine density and arborization of dendrites are directly regulated by miR-132, miR-134 and miR-9 [20–24, 124, 125]. miR-132 is significantly increased in the hippocampus of experimental mice undergoing seizure and its inhibition has been shown to increase neuronal survival and reduce seizure frequency [126, 127]. Upregulation of miR-134 has been identified in resected hippocampal and neocortical tissue of patients with treatment-resistant temporal-lobe epilepsy [128]. This was also observed in a number of animal models where inhibition of miR-134 was shown to reduce seizure occurrence and increase spine volume in hippocampal neurons [128–130]. Neuronal potassium channel expression is regulated by miR-92a and miR-324. miR-92a has been shown to be increased in temporal lobe epilepsy patients, and in animal models of epilepsy inhibition of miR-324 delays the onset of spontaneous seizures [131, 132]. Finally, the Ca^{2+} extruding pump ATP2B4 and the sodium-potassium-chloride transporter NKCC1 are regulated by miR-129 and miR-101a respectively. miR-129 is increased in temporal lobe epilepsy patients and inhibition of miR-1219 and miR-101a have been shown to reduce hyperexcitability in animal models of epilepsy [133, 134].

Recently, serum from two independent cohorts of temporal-lobe epilepsy patients have revealed increased levels of three 5′tRFS, 5′AlaTGC, 5′GluCTC and 5′GlyGCC. These tRFs were detected in resected hippocampal and cortical tissue and were not associated with any disease related lesions. Furthermore, these fragments were detected in primary mouse hippocampal neurons and their expression was shown to be activity-related [135].

5. ncRNA as a biomarker for disease

5.1 ncRNA biomarkers in Parkinson's disease

A number of candidate miRNAs have been identified in plasma from PD patients by microarray, and validation in an independent cohort revealed the expression of miR-1826/miR-450b-3p, miR-626 and miR-505 were significantly different between control and PD subjects [136]. In a larger study, miRNAs known to be expressed in the CNS and involved in neuronal regulation were identified in the plasma of PD patients. The expression of miR-137 was increases and expression of miR-124 was decreased in PD patients compared with controls; however, there was no relation between these alterations and the severity of disease [137]. Using sequencing technologies a number of studies have identified miRNA candidates as biomarkers for PD. Subsequent validation by RT-PCR determined that miR-195 was increased and miR-185, miR-15b, miR-221, miR-181a, miR-141, miR-214, miR-146b-5p, miR-193-3p, miR-29c, miR-146a, miR-214 and miR-221 were decreased in PD patients [138–140]. Finally, one study identified differential expression of miR-1-3p, miR-22-5p and miR-29a-3p in the whole blood of PD patients using PCR [141]. It is important to note here that no miRNA has yet been identified as a biomarker for PD in two independent studies.

A number of independent studies have identified *Ang* variants in PD [78, 79], however the investigation of tsRNA as a biomarker for the disease is in its infancy. Using deep sequencing analysis of postmortem tissue Pantano et al. identified that tsRNA clusters can accurately differentiate between control, PD patients at premotor and motor stages of the disease [80]. Furthermore, in a small study sex-specific tsRNA differences were reported in the prefrontal cortex, cerebrospinal fluid and serum of PD patients [81].

5.2 miRNA biomarkers in Alzheimer's disease

In 2014, two independent studies reported a downregulation of miR-125b in the serum of AD patients and Tan et al. correlated this with cognitive decline [142, 143]. Interestingly, a number of studies have also identified multiple miRNA panels that demonstrate diagnostic value. In a small cohort of patients a group of 7 miRNAs were shown to be differentially expressed in the plasma of AD patients [144]. In a larger study, next-generation sequencing identified 140 differentially expressed miRNAs. Subsequent validation studies using RT-PCR in a cohort of 202 patient samples demonstrated a 12-miRNA signature to differentiate between AD and control samples to a high degree of sensitivity [145]. Finally, next-generation sequencing of exosomes extracted from the blood revealed a 16-miRNA signature differentially expressed in AD patients. Validated by RT-PCR and combined with known risk factors such as age, sex and apolipoprotein ε4 allele status provided prognosis with high sensitivity [146].

5.3 miRNA biomarkers in stroke

The multi-targeting potential of miRNAs places them in a powerful position in the diagnosis and prognosis of heterogeneous conditions such as stroke, where early diagnosis has significant implications for prognosis. A number of miRNAs have been shown to demonstrate diagnostic and prognostic value in acute stroke, and a recent systemic review and bioinformatic analysis has highlighted and identified the most promising candidates [147]. miR-16 has been identified as significantly upregulated in the plasma of acute ischemic stroke (AIS) patients, and upregulation of miR-16 is associated with poorer prognosis (mRS 3–6) [148, 149]. Independent studies have identified the downregulation of miR-126 in plasma from AIS patients as a biomarker of disease severity. Circulating levels of miR-126 negatively correlated with pro-inflammatory cytokine levels and National Institute of Health Stroke Scale (NIHSS) scores [150–152]. Similarly, downregulation of circulating miR-355 has also been reported as having high sensitivity as a biomarker of acute ischaemic stroke and to correlate negatively with NIHSS scores in AIS patients [153].

Upregulation of miR-130a has been reported as a potential biomarker in the diagnosis of brain oedema and prognosis in haemorrhagic stroke, positively correlating with NIHSS and mRS scores [154]. Moreover, antagonism of miR-130a expression in *in vivo* and *in vitro* models of ischaemia demonstrated attenuation of brain oedema and reduced blood-brain barrier permeability.

5.4 ncRNA biomarkers in amyolateral sclerosis

In a series of studies Freischmidt et al. identified a number of miRNAs differentially expressed in the serum of familial (miR-143-5p/3p, miR-132-5p/3p and miR-574-5p/3p) and sporadic (miR-1234-3p and miR-1825) ALS, noting that miRNA targets in familial ALS were TDP-43 binding RNAs and that the miRNA signature in sporadic ALS was highly heterogeneous [155, 156]. A subsequent study determined increased miR-374b-5p, and decreased miR-206 and miR-143-3p in sporadic ALS patient serum [157]. Finally, increased expression of miR-424 and miR-206 in sporadic ALS patient plasma has been shown to correlate with clinical deterioration over time [111].

Recent work has identified 5'tiRNA$^{Val-CAC}$ as a potential biomarker for ALS. This tiRNA was found to be increased in the spinal cord of SOD1^{G93A} mice and is significantly increased in the serum of patients with slow progressing ALS [120].

5.5 ncRNA biomarkers in epilepsy

Circulating miRNAs have been found to be dysregulated in the serum of epilepsy patients compared with healthy controls. Validation experiments identified an upregulation of let-7d-5p, miR-106b-5p, miR-130a-3p and miR-146a-5p, and a downregulation of miR-15a-5p and miR-194-5p. The highest diagnostic value was found in the upregulated miR-106b-5p [158]. Further studies also revealed miRNAs differentially expressed in treatment-resistant compared to treatment-responsive and control samples. The expression of miR-194-5p, miR-301a-3p, miR-30b-5p, miR-342-5p and miR-4446-3p were altered in drug-resistant epilepsy serum samples, with miR-301a-3p showing the highest sensitivity [159]. Finally, sequencing analysis and RT-qPCR validation identified miR-27a-3p, miR-328-3p and miR-654-3p as differentially expressed in the plasma of epilepsy patients compared to control. Importantly, these miRNAs were detected using a prototype point-of-care device that would greatly improve diagnostic capability in-clinic [160].

Recent sequencing analysis has identified three circulating tRFs that are increased in the plasma of epilepsy patients. The differential expression of 5′AlaTGC, 5′GluCTC and 5′GlyGCC was validated by RT-qPCR in an independent cohort and detected in resected hippocampal and cortical tissue indicating a possible source. Finally, the generation and release of these tRFs was shown to be activity-related in mouse hippocampal neuronal cultures [135].

6. ncRNA as a therapeutic target

The direct involvement of miRNA and tsRNA in normal cellular activity, their dysregulation during disease pathogenesis and ability to target multiple genes within a particular pathway have made ncRNA an attractive and viable therapeutic target for the treatment of many neurological diseases. Therapeutic intervention strategies include the inhibition of overexpressed ncRNA and the restoration of repressed ncRNA. Small interfering RNA (siRNA) and antisense oligonucleotides (ASO) are the most common methods of miRNA inhibition. siRNA are short (20–25 nts) double-stranded RNA molecules that use the RNA interference RISC pathway to degrade target RNA. ASOs, also known as antimiRs or antagomiRs, are short single stranded oligonucleotides that hybridize with the target RNA and sterically interfere with its functionality. Recent advancements include the development of locked nucleic acid technology that increases the stability of ASO and siRNA [161]. The restoration miRNA expression suppressed in a given pathology through the delivery of synthetic double-stranded miRNA mimics, designed to mimic endogenous miRNAs, so far has primarily been used in gain-of-function studies to elucidate miRNA functions and mechanisms [98].

While a considerable amount of progress has been made with a number of miRNAs entering clinical trials, the development of RNA-based therapeutics has not been without issue. Double- and single-stranded RNA are recognized by the immune system, particularly the Toll-like receptors. To combat this, 2'O-methylation and the neutralization of RNA molecules significantly reduces the immunogenicity of RNA-based therapeutics [162–164]. Delivery systems to aid passage across the cell membrane and the targeting of specific organs and cells types have also been developed. Lipid and metal-based nanoparticles as well as polymer vectors such as polyethylene imine, polylactic-co-glycolic acid and poly-amidoamine have improved the delivery of RNA-based therapeutics [165]. Furthermore, artificial manipulation of miRNAs with the delivery of miRNA mimics *in vivo* is associated with difficult to predict off-target non-specific and unintended alterations in gene expression, and toxicity, off-setting potential for therapeutic efficacy [166].

To date the Federal Drug Administration and the European Medicines Agency have approved a number of RNA-based therapeutics [167]. Notably the 18-mer ASO Nusinersen is an intrathecal administered therapeutic for the treatment of spinal muscular atrophy. Phase II and III clinical trials are also ongoing for RNA-based therapeutics for the treatment of Huntington's disease [165].

7. Conclusions

Over the past two decades research into miRNA and, more recently, tsRNA has demonstrated the integral role that these ncRNA play in cellular function and dysfunction. This has been particularly apparent in diseases of the central nervous system. Advancements in sequencing technologies and other RNA detection methods have highlighted their utility as biomarkers and the potential for disease stratification. RNA-based therapeutic intervention has shown great promise in areas with limited treatment options. Rapid improvements in the delivery and immunoreactivity of these treatments and the increasing number of clinical trials involving RNA-based therapeutics is encouraging.

Conflict of interest

The authors declare no conflict of interest.

Author details

Steven G. Fagan and Shona Pfeiffer*
Royal College of Surgeons in Ireland, Dublin, Ireland

*Address all correspondence to: shonapfeiffer@rcsi.com

References

[1] Djebali S, Davis CA, Merkel A, Dobin A, Lassmann T, Mortazavi A, et al. Landscape of transcription in human cells. Nature. 2012;**489**(7414):101-108

[2] Dunham I, Kundaje A, Aldred SF, Collins PJ, Davis CA, Doyle F, et al. An integrated encyclopedia of DNA elements in the human genome. Nature. 2012;**489**(7414):57-74

[3] Mercer TR, Dinger ME, Mattick JS. Long non-coding RNAs: Insights into functions. Nature Reviews. Genetics. 2009;**10**(3):155-159

[4] Zhang P, Wu W, Chen Q, Chen M. Non-coding RNAs and their integrated networks. Journal of Integrative Bioinformatics. 2019;**16**(3):20190027

[5] Giraldez AJ, Cinalli RM, Glasner ME, Enright AJ, Thomson JM, Baskerville S, et al. MicroRNAs regulate brain morphogenesis in Zebrafish. Science. 2005;**308**(5723):833-838

[6] Davis TH, Cuellar TL, Koch SM, Barker AJ, Harfe BD, McManus MT, et al. Conditional loss of Dicer disrupts cellular and tissue morphogenesis in the cortex and hippocampus. The Journal of Neuroscience. 2008;**28**(17):4322-4330

[7] Kawase-Koga Y, Otaegi G, Sun T. Different timings of Dicer deletion affect neurogenesis and gliogenesis in the developing mouse central nervous system. Developmental Dynamics. 2009;**238**(11):2800-2812

[8] Liu C, Teng Z-Q, Santistevan NJ, Szulwach KE, Guo W, Jin P, et al. Epigenetic regulation of miR-184 by MBD1 governs neural stem cell proliferation and differentiation. Cell Stem Cell. 2010;**6**(5):433-444

[9] Liu C, Teng Z-Q, McQuate AL, Jobe EM, Christ CC, von Hoyningen-Huene SJ, et al. An epigenetic feedback regulatory loop involving microRNA-195 and MBD1 governs neural stem cell differentiation. PLoS One. 2013;**8**(1):e51436-e

[10] Brett JO, Renault VM, Rafalski VA, Webb AE, Brunet A. The microRNA cluster miR-106b~25 regulates adult neural stem/progenitor cell proliferation and neuronal differentiation. Aging (Albany NY). 2011;**3**(2):108-124

[11] Yang D, Li T, Wang Y, Tang Y, Cui H, Tang Y, et al. miR-132 regulates the differentiation of dopamine neurons by directly targeting Nurr1 expression. Journal of Cell Science. 2012;**125**(7): 1673-1682

[12] Kim J, Inoue K, Ishii J, Vanti WB, Voronov SV, Murchison E, et al. A MicroRNA feedback circuit in midbrain dopamine neurons. Science (New York, N.Y.). 2007;**317**(5842):1220-1224

[13] He M, Liu Y, Wang X, Zhang MQ, Hannon GJ, Huang ZJ. Cell-type-based analysis of microRNA profiles in the mouse brain. Neuron. 2012;**73**(1):35-48

[14] de Chevigny A, Coré N, Follert P, Gaudin M, Barbry P, Béclin C, et al. miR-7a regulation of Pax6 controls spatial origin of forebrain dopaminergic neurons. Nature Neuroscience. 2012;**15**(8):1120-1126

[15] Rago L, Beattie R, Taylor V, Winter J. miR379-410 cluster miRNAs regulate neurogenesis and neuronal migration by fine-tuning N-cadherin. The EMBO Journal. 2014;**33**(8):906-920

[16] Luikart BW, Bensen AL, Washburn EK, Perederiy JV, Su KG, Li Y, et al. miR-132 mediates the integration of newborn neurons into the adult dentate gyrus. PLoS One. 2011;**6**(5):e19077-e

[17] Vo N, Klein ME, Varlamova O, Keller DM, Yamamoto T, Goodman RH,

et al. A cAMP-response element binding protein-induced microRNA regulates neuronal morphogenesis. Proceedings of the National Academy of Sciences of the United States of America. 2005; **102**(45):16426-16431

[18] Zhang Y, Ueno Y, Liu XS, Buller B, Wang X, Chopp M, et al. The MicroRNA-17-92 cluster enhances axonal outgrowth in embryonic cortical neurons. The Journal of Neuroscience. 2013;**33**(16):6885-6894

[19] Dajas-Bailador F, Bonev B, Garcez P, Stanley P, Guillemot F, Papalopulu N. microRNA-9 regulates axon extension and branching by targeting Map1b in mouse cortical neurons. Nature Neuroscience. 2012;**15**(5):697-699

[20] Giusti SA, Vogl AM, Brockmann MM, Vercelli CA, Rein ML, Trümbach D, et al. MicroRNA-9 controls dendritic development by targeting REST. eLife. 2014;**3**:e02755

[21] Pathania M, Torres-Reveron J, Yan L, Kimura T, Lin TV, Gordon V, et al. miR-132 enhances dendritic morphogenesis, spine density, synaptic integration, and survival of newborn olfactory bulb neurons. PLoS One. 2012;**7**(5):e38174

[22] Magill ST, Cambronne XA, Luikart BW, Lioy DT, Leighton BH, Westbrook GL, et al. microRNA-132 regulates dendritic growth and arborization of newborn neurons in the adult hippocampus. Proceedings of the National Academy of Sciences of the United States of America. 2010;**107**(47):20382-20387

[23] Jasińska M, Miłek J, Cymerman IA, Łęski S, Kaczmarek L, Dziembowska M. miR-132 regulates dendritic spine structure by direct targeting of matrix metalloproteinase 9 mRNA. Molecular Neurobiology. 2016;**53**(7):4701-4712

[24] Dhar M, Zhu M, Impey S, Lambert TJ, Bland T, Karatsoreos IN, et al. Leptin induces hippocampal synaptogenesis via CREB-regulated microRNA-132 suppression of p250GAP. Molecular Endocrinology. 2014;**28**(7): 1073-1087

[25] Karr J, Vagin V, Chen K, Ganesan S, Olenkina O, Gvozdev V, et al. Regulation of glutamate receptor subunit availability by microRNAs. The Journal of Cell Biology. 2009;**185**(4):685-697

[26] Wang RY, Phang RZ, Hsu PH, Wang WH, Huang HT, Liu IY. In vivo knockdown of hippocampal miR-132 expression impairs memory acquisition of trace fear conditioning. Hippocampus. 2013;**23**(7):625-633

[27] Skaper SD, Facci L, Zusso M, Giusti P. An inflammation-centric view of neurological disease: Beyond the neuron. Frontiers in Cellular Neuroscience. 2018;**12**:72

[28] Jovičić A, Roshan R, Moisoi N, Pradervand S, Moser R, Pillai B, et al. Comprehensive expression analyses of neural cell-type-specific miRNAs identify new determinants of the specification and maintenance of neuronal phenotypes. The Journal of Neuroscience. 2013;**33**(12):5127-5137

[29] Freilich RW, Woodbury ME, Ikezu T. Integrated expression profiles of mRNA and miRNA in polarized primary murine microglia. PLoS One. 2013;**8**(11):e79416

[30] Su W, Hopkins S, Nesser NK, Sopher B, Silvestroni A, Ammanuel S, et al. The p53 transcription factor modulates microglia behavior through microRNA-dependent regulation of c-Maf. Journal of Immunology. 2014; **192**(1):358-366

[31] Li YY, Cui JG, Dua P, Pogue AI, Bhattacharjee S, Lukiw WJ. Differential expression of miRNA-146a-regulated inflammatory genes in human primary neural, astroglial and microglial cells.

Neuroscience Letters. 2011;**499**(2): 109-113

[32] Ma C, Li Y, Li M, Deng G, Wu X, Zeng J, et al. microRNA-124 negatively regulates TLR signaling in alveolar macrophages in response to mycobacterial infection. Molecular Immunology. 2014;**62**(1):150-158

[33] Ponomarev ED, Veremeyko T, Barteneva N, Krichevsky AM, Weiner HL. MicroRNA-124 promotes microglia quiescence and suppresses EAE by deactivating macrophages via the C/EBP-alpha-PU.1 pathway. Nature Medicine. 2011;**17**(1):64-70

[34] Zhu H, Xie R, Liu X, Shou J, Gu W, Gu S, et al. MicroRNA-494 improves functional recovery and inhibits apoptosis by modulating PTEN/AKT/mTOR pathway in rats after spinal cord injury. Biomedicine & Pharmacotherapy. 2017;**92**:879-887

[35] Lv X, Liang J, Wang Z. MiR-21-5p reduces apoptosis and inflammation in rats with spinal cord injury through PI3K/AKT pathway. Panminerva Med. 2020. DOI: 10.23736/S0031-0808.20.03974-9

[36] Xiao X, Li W, Rong D, Xu Z, Zhang Z, Ye H, Xie L, Wu Y, Zhang Y, Wang X. Human umbilical cord mesenchymal stem cells-derived extracellular vesicles facilitate the repair of spinal cord injury via the miR-29b-3p/PTEN/Akt/mTOR axis. Cell Death Discov. 2021;**7**(1):212

[37] Liu W, Chen X, Zhang Y. Effects of microRNA-21 and microRNA-24 inhibitors on neuronal apoptosis in ischemic stroke. Am J Transl Res. 2016;**8**(7):3179-3187

[38] Yin KJ, Deng Z, Huang H, Hamblin M, Xie C, Zhang J, Chen YE. miR-497 regulates neuronal death in mouse brain after transient focal cerebral ischemia. Neurobiol Dis. 2010;**38**(1):17-26

[39] Cimmino A, Calin GA, Fabbri M, et al. miR-15 and miR-16 induce apoptosis by targeting BCL2 [published correction appears in Proc Natl Acad Sci U S A. 2006 Feb 14;103(7):2464]. Proc Natl Acad Sci U S A. 2005;**102**(39): 13944-13949

[40] Moon J, Xu L, Giffard RG. Inhibition of microRNA-181 Reduces Forebrain Ischemia-Induced Neuronal Loss. J Cereb Blood Flow Metab. 2013;**33**(12):1976-1982

[41] Li P, Shen M, Gao F, Wu J, Zhang J, Teng F, et al. An antagomir to microRNA-106b-5p ameliorates cerebral ischemia and reperfusion injury in rats via inhibiting apoptosis and oxidative stress. Molecular Neurobiology. 2017;**54**(4):2901-2921

[42] Walker SC, Engelke DR. Ribonuclease P: The evolution of an ancient RNA enzyme. Critical Reviews in Biochemistry and Molecular Biology. 2006;**41**(2):77-102

[43] Phizicky EM, Hopper AK. tRNA biology charges to the front. Genes & Development. 2010;**24**(17):1832-1860

[44] Phizicky EM, Hopper AK. tRNA processing, modification, and subcellular dynamics: Past, present, and future. RNA. 2015;**21**(4):483-485

[45] Wellner K, Betat H, Mörl M. A tRNA's fate is decided at its 3′ end: Collaborative actions of CCA-adding enzyme and RNases involved in tRNA processing and degradation. Biochimica et Biophysica Acta. Gene Regulatory Mechanisms. 2018;**1861**(4):433-441

[46] Wilusz JE, Whipple JM, Phizicky EM, Sharp PA. tRNAs marked with CCACCA are targeted for degradation. Science. 2011;**334**(6057): 817-821

[47] Giegé R, Jühling F, Pütz J, Stadler P, Sauter C, Florentz C. Structure of

transfer RNAs: Similarity and variability. Wiley Interdisciplinary Reviews: RNA. 2012;**3**(1):37-61

[48] Boccaletto P, Machnicka MA, Purta E, Piatkowski P, Baginski B, Wirecki TK, et al. MODOMICS: A database of RNA modification pathways. 2017 update. Nucleic Acids Research. 2018;**46**(D1):D303-D3d7

[49] Motorin Y, Helm M. tRNA stabilization by modified nucleotides. Biochemistry. 2010;**49**(24):4934-4944

[50] Helm M. Post-transcriptional nucleotide modification and alternative folding of RNA. Nucleic Acids Research. 2006;**34**(2):721-733

[51] Yamasaki S, Ivanov P, Hu GF, Anderson P. Angiogenin cleaves tRNA and promotes stress-induced translational repression. The Journal of Cell Biology. 2009;**185**(1):35-42

[52] Nakamura M, Yamabe H, Osawa H, Nakamura N, Shimada M, Kumasaka R, et al. Hypoxic conditions stimulate the production of angiogenin and vascular endothelial growth factor by human renal proximal tubular epithelial cells in culture. Nephrology, Dialysis, Transplantation. 2006;**21**(6):1489-1495

[53] Saikia M, Jobava R, Parisien M, Putnam A, Krokowski D, Gao XH, et al. Angiogenin-cleaved tRNA halves interact with cytochrome c, protecting cells from apoptosis during osmotic stress. Molecular and Cellular Biology. 2014;**34**(13):2450-2463

[54] Emara MM, Ivanov P, Hickman T, Dawra N, Tisdale S, Kedersha N, et al. Angiogenin-induced tRNA-derived stress-induced RNAs promote stress-induced stress granule assembly. The Journal of Biological Chemistry. 2010;**285**(14):10959-10968

[55] Elkordy A, Rashad S, Shehabeldeen H, Mishima E, Niizuma K, Abe T, et al. tiRNAs as a novel biomarker for cell damage assessment in in vitro ischemia-reperfusion model in rat neuronal PC12 cells. Brain Research. 2019;**1714**:8-17

[56] Elkordy A, Mishima E, Niizuma K, Akiyama Y, Fujimura M, Tominaga T, et al. Stress-induced tRNA cleavage and tiRNA generation in rat neuronal PC12 cells. Journal of Neurochemistry. 2018;**146**(5):560-569

[57] Kumar P, Kuscu C, Dutta A. Biogenesis and function of transfer RNA-related fragments (tRFs). Trends in Biochemical Sciences. 2016;**41**(8):679-689

[58] Fagan SG, Helm M, Prehn JHM. tRNA-derived fragments: A new class of non-coding RNA with key roles in nervous system function and dysfunction. Progress in Neurobiology. 2021;**205**:102118

[59] Kumar P, Anaya J, Mudunuri SB, Dutta A. Meta-analysis of tRNA derived RNA fragments reveals that they are evolutionarily conserved and associate with AGO proteins to recognize specific RNA targets. BMC Biology. 2014;**12**:78

[60] Karaiskos S, Naqvi AS, Swanson KE, Grigoriev A. Age-driven modulation of tRNA-derived fragments in Drosophila and their potential targets. Biology Direct. 2015;**10**:51

[61] Merrick WC, Pavitt GD. Protein synthesis initiation in eukaryotic cells. Cold Spring Harbor Perspectives in Biology. 2018;**10**:a033092

[62] Protter DSW, Parker R. Principles and properties of stress granules. Trends in Cell Biology. 2016;**26**(9):668-679

[63] Lyons SM, Achorn C, Kedersha NL, Anderson PJ, Ivanov P. YB-1 regulates tiRNA-induced stress granule formation but not translational repression. Nucleic Acids Research. 2016;**44**(14):6949-6960

[64] Gebetsberger J, Zywicki M, Künzi A, Polacek N. tRNA-derived fragments target the ribosome and function as regulatory non-coding RNA in Haloferax volcanii. Archaea. 2012;**2012**:260909

[65] Gebetsberger J, Wyss L, Mleczko AM, Reuther J, Polacek N. A tRNA-derived fragment competes with mRNA for ribosome binding and regulates translation during stress. RNA Biology. 2017;**14**(10):1364-1373

[66] Kuscu C, Kumar P, Kiran M, Su Z, Malik A, Dutta A. tRNA fragments (tRFs) guide Ago to regulate gene expression post-transcriptionally in a Dicer-independent manner. RNA (New York, NY). 2018;**24**(8):1093-1105

[67] Blanco S, Dietmann S, Flores JV, Hussain S, Kutter C, Humphreys P, et al. Aberrant methylation of tRNAs links cellular stress to neuro-developmental disorders. The EMBO Journal. 2014;**33**(18):2020-2039

[68] Hanada T, Weitzer S, Mair B, Bernreuther C, Wainger BJ, Ichida J, et al. CLP1 links tRNA metabolism to progressive motor-neuron loss. Nature. 2013;**495**(7442):474-480

[69] Zhang X, He X, Liu C, Liu J, Hu Q, Pan T, et al. IL-4 inhibits the biogenesis of an epigenetically suppressive PIWI-interacting RNA to upregulate CD1a molecules on monocytes/dendritic cells. Journal of Immunology. 2016;**196**(4): 1591-1603

[70] Green JA, Ansari MY, Ball HC, Haqqi TM. tRNA-derived fragments (tRFs) regulate post-transcriptional gene expression via AGO-dependent mechanism in IL-1β stimulated chondrocytes. Osteoarthritis and Cartilage. 2020;**28**(8):1102-1110

[71] Wang Z, Xiang L, Shao J, Yuan Z. The 3' CCACCA sequence of tRNAAla(UGC) is the motif that is important in inducing Th1-like immune response, and this motif can be recognized by Toll-like receptor 3. Clinical and Vaccine Immunology. 2006;**13**(7):733-739

[72] Berwick DC, Heaton GR, Azeggagh S, Harvey K. LRRK2 Biology from structure to dysfunction: Research progresses, but the themes remain the same. Molecular Neurodegeneration. 2019;**14**(1):49

[73] Cho HJ, Liu G, Jin SM, Parisiadou L, Xie C, Yu J, et al. MicroRNA-205 regulates the expression of Parkinson's disease-related leucine-rich repeat kinase 2 protein. Human Molecular Genetics. 2013;**22**(3):608-620

[74] Gehrke S, Imai Y, Sokol N, Lu B. Pathogenic LRRK2 negatively regulates microRNA-mediated translational repression. Nature. 2010;**466**(7306): 637-641

[75] Doxakis E. Post-transcriptional regulation of alpha-synuclein expression by mir-7 and mir-153. The Journal of Biological Chemistry. 2010;**285**(17):12726-12734

[76] Wang G, van der Walt JM, Mayhew G, Li YJ, Züchner S, Scott WK, et al. Variation in the miRNA-433 binding site of FGF20 confers risk for Parkinson disease by overexpression of alpha-synuclein. American Journal of Human Genetics. 2008;**82**(2):283-289

[77] Gong X, Wang H, Ye Y, Shu Y, Deng Y, He X, et al. miR-124 regulates cell apoptosis and autophagy in dopaminergic neurons and protects them by regulating AMPK/mTOR pathway in Parkinson's disease. American Journal of Translational Research. 2016;**8**(5):2127-2137

[78] Rayaprolu S, Soto-Ortolaza A, Rademakers R, Uitti RJ, Wszolek ZK, Ross OA. Angiogenin variation and Parkinson disease. Annals of Neurology. 2012;**71**(5):725-728

[79] van Es MA, Schelhaas HJ, van Vught PW, Ticozzi N, Andersen PM, Groen EJ, et al. Angiogenin variants in Parkinson disease and amyotrophic lateral sclerosis. Annals of Neurology. 2011;**70**(6):964-973

[80] Pantano L, Friedländer MR, Escaramís G, Lizano E, Pallarès-Albanell J, Ferrer I, et al. Specific small-RNA signatures in the amygdala at premotor and motor stages of Parkinson's disease revealed by deep sequencing analysis. Bioinformatics. 2016;**32**(5):673-681

[81] Magee R, Londin E, Rigoutsos I. TRNA-derived fragments as sex-dependent circulating candidate biomarkers for Parkinson's disease. Parkinsonism & Related Disorders. 2019;**65**:203-209

[82] Denk J, Boelmans K, Siegismund C, Lassner D, Arlt S, Jahn H. MicroRNA profiling of CSF reveals potential biomarkers to detect Alzheimer's disease. PLoS One. 2015;**10**(5):e0126423

[83] Tan L, Yu JT, Tan MS, Liu QY, Wang HF, Zhang W, et al. Genome-wide serum microRNA expression profiling identifies serum biomarkers for Alzheimer's disease. Journal of Alzheimer's Disease. 2014;**40**(4): 1017-1027

[84] Cogswell JP, Ward J, Taylor IA, Waters M, Shi Y, Cannon B, et al. Identification of miRNA changes in Alzheimer's disease brain and CSF yields putative biomarkers and insights into disease pathways. Journal of Alzheimer's Disease. 2008;**14**(1):27-41

[85] Zhao Y, Pogue AI, Lukiw WJ. MicroRNA (miRNA) signaling in the human CNS in sporadic Alzheimer's disease (AD)-novel and unique pathological features. International Journal of Molecular Sciences. 2015;**16**(12):30105-30116

[86] Smith P, Al Hashimi A, Girard J, Delay C, Hébert SS. In vivo regulation of amyloid precursor protein neuronal splicing by microRNAs. Journal of Neurochemistry. 2011;**116**(2):240-247

[87] Donev R, Newall A, Thome J, Sheer D. A role for SC35 and hnRNPA1 in the determination of amyloid precursor protein isoforms. Molecular Psychiatry. 2007;**12**(7):681-690

[88] Hu YK, Wang X, Li L, Du YH, Ye HT, Li CY. MicroRNA-98 induces an Alzheimer's disease-like disturbance by targeting insulin-like growth factor 1. Neuroscience Bulletin. 2013;**29**(6):745-751

[89] Absalon S, Kochanek DM, Raghavan V, Krichevsky AM. MiR-26b, upregulated in Alzheimer's disease, activates cell cycle entry, tau-phosphorylation, and apoptosis in postmitotic neurons. The Journal of Neuroscience. 2013;**33**(37):14645-14659

[90] Dickson JR, Kruse C, Montagna DR, Finsen B, Wolfe MS. Alternative polyadenylation and miR-34 family members regulate tau expression. Journal of Neurochemistry. 2013;**127**(6):739-749

[91] Jayadev S, Case A, Alajajian B, Eastman AJ, Möller T, Garden GA. Presenilin 2 influences miR146 level and activity in microglia. Journal of Neurochemistry. 2013;**127**(5):592-599

[92] Malpetti M, Kievit RA, Passamonti L, Jones PS, Tsvetanov KA, Rittman T, et al. Microglial activation and tau burden predict cognitive decline in Alzheimer's disease. Brain. 2020;**143**(5):1588-1602

[93] Gagliardi S, Davin A, Bini P, Sinforiani E, Poloni TE, Polito L, et al. A novel nonsense angiogenin mutation is associated with Alzheimer disease. Alzheimer Disease and Associated Disorders. 2019;**33**(2):163-165

[94] Dirnagl U, Iadecola C, Moskowitz MA. Pathobiology of ischaemic stroke: An integrated view.

Trends in Neurosciences. 1999;**22**(9):391-397

[95] Belov Kirdajova D, Kriska J, Tureckova J, Anderova M. Ischemia-triggered glutamate excitotoxicity from the perspective of glial cells. Frontiers in Cellular Neuroscience. 2020;**14**:51

[96] Yang ZB, Zhang Z, Li TB, Lou Z, Li SY, Yang H, et al. Up-regulation of brain-enriched miR-107 promotes excitatory neurotoxicity through down-regulation of glutamate transporter-1 expression following ischaemic stroke. Clinical Science (London, England). 2014;**127**(12):679-689

[97] Chan SY, Loscalzo J. MicroRNA-210: A unique and pleiotropic hypoxamir. Cell Cycle. 2010;**9**(6):1072-1083

[98] Pfeiffer S, Tomascova A, Mamrak U, Haunsberger SJ, Connolly NMC, Resler A, et al. AMPK-regulated miRNA-210-3p is activated during ischaemic neuronal injury and modulates PI3K-p70S6K signalling. Journal of Neurochemistry. 2021;**159**(4):710-728

[99] Majdi A, Mahmoudi J, Sadigh-Eteghad S, Farhoudi M, Shotorbani SS. The interplay of microRNAs and post-ischemic glutamate excitotoxicity: An emergent research field in stroke medicine. Neurological Sciences. 2016;**37**(11):1765-1771

[100] Harraz MM, Eacker SM, Wang X, Dawson TM, Dawson VL. MicroRNA-223 is neuroprotective by targeting glutamate receptors. Proceedings of the National Academy of Sciences of the United States of America. 2012;**109**(46): 18962-18967

[101] Sun Y, Luo ZM, Guo XM, Su DF, Liu X. An updated role of microRNA-124 in central nervous system disorders: A review. Frontiers in Cellular Neuroscience. 2015;**9**:193

[102] Shi Y, Tian T, Cai EL, Yang C, Yang X. Corrigendum: miR-124 alleviates ischemic stroke-induced neuronal death by targeting DAPK1 in mice. Frontiers in Neuroscience. 2021;**15**:745087

[103] Sun Y, Gui H, Li Q, Luo ZM, Zheng MJ, Duan JL, et al. MicroRNA-124 protects neurons against apoptosis in cerebral ischemic stroke. CNS Neuroscience & Therapeutics. 2013;**19**(10):813-819

[104] Zhang L, Dong LY, Li YJ, Hong Z, Wei WS. The microRNA miR-181c controls microglia-mediated neuronal apoptosis by suppressing tumor necrosis factor. Journal of Neuroinflammation. 2012;**9**:211

[105] Sato K, Rashad S, Niizuma K, Tominaga T. Stress induced tRNA halves (tiRNAs) as biomarkers for stroke and stroke therapy; Pre-clinical Study. Neuroscience. 2020;**434**:44-54

[106] Li J, Wang Y. Blood biomarkers in minor stroke and transient ischemic attack. Neuroscience Bulletin. 2016;**32**(5):463-468

[107] Turner MR, Hardiman O, Benatar M, Brooks BR, Chio A, de Carvalho M, et al. Controversies and priorities in amyotrophic lateral sclerosis. Lancet Neurology. 2013;**12**(3):310-322

[108] Hardiman O, Al-Chalabi A, Chio A, Corr EM, Logroscino G, Robberecht W, et al. Amyotrophic lateral sclerosis. Nature Reviews Disease Primers. 2017;**3**(1):17071

[109] Renton AE, Chiò A, Traynor BJ. State of play in amyotrophic lateral sclerosis genetics. Nature Neuroscience. 2014;**17**(1):17-23

[110] Matamala JM, Arias-Carrasco R, Sanchez C, Uhrig M, Bargsted L,

Matus S, et al. Genome-wide circulating microRNA expression profiling reveals potential biomarkers for amyotrophic lateral sclerosis. Neurobiology of Aging. 2018;**64**:123-138

[111] de Andrade HM, de Albuquerque M, Avansini SH, de Cristiane SRC, Dogini DB, Nucci A, et al. MicroRNAs-424 and 206 are potential prognostic markers in spinal onset amyotrophic lateral sclerosis. Journal of the Neurological Sciences. 2016;**368**:19-24

[112] Pegoraro V, Merico A, Angelini C. Micro-RNAs in ALS muscle: Differences in gender, age at onset and disease duration. Journal of the Neurological Sciences. 2017;**380**:58-63

[113] Tasca E, Pegoraro V, Merico A, Angelini C. Circulating microRNAs as biomarkers of muscle differentiation and atrophy in ALS. Clinical Neuropathology. 2016;**35**(1):22-30

[114] Koval ED, Shaner C, Zhang P, du Maine X, Fischer K, Tay J, et al. Method for widespread microRNA-155 inhibition prolongs survival in ALS-model mice. Human Molecular Genetics. 2013;**22**(20):4127-4135

[115] Yamakuchi M, Ferlito M, Lowenstein CJ. miR-34a repression of SIRT1 regulates apoptosis. Proceedings of the National Academy of Sciences of the United States of America. 2008;**105**(36):13421-13426

[116] Rizzuti M, Filosa G, Melzi V, Calandriello L, Dioni L, Bollati V, et al. MicroRNA expression analysis identifies a subset of downregulated miRNAs in ALS motor neuron progenitors. Scientific Reports. 2018;**8**(1):10105

[117] Wu D, Yu W, Kishikawa H, Folkerth RD, Iafrate AJ, Shen Y, et al. Angiogenin loss-of-function mutations in amyotrophic lateral sclerosis. Annals of Neurology. 2007;**62**(6):609-617

[118] Greenway MJ, Andersen PM, Russ C, Ennis S, Cashman S, Donaghy C, et al. ANG mutations segregate with familial and 'sporadic' amyotrophic lateral sclerosis. Nature Genetics. 2006;**38**(4):411-413

[119] Crabtree B, Thiyagarajan N, Prior SH, Wilson P, Iyer S, Ferns T, et al. Characterization of human angiogenin variants implicated in amyotrophic lateral sclerosis. Biochemistry. 2007;**46**(42):11810-11818

[120] Hogg MC, Rayner M, Susdalzew S, Monsefi N, Crivello M, Woods I, et al. 5′ValCAC tRNA fragment generated as part of a protective angiogenin response provides prognostic value in amyotrophic lateral sclerosis. Brain Communications. 2020;**2**(2):fcaa138

[121] Global, regional, and national burden of epilepsy, 1990-2016: A systematic analysis for the Global Burden of Disease Study 2016. Lancet Neurology. 2019;**18**(4):357-375

[122] Pernice HF, Schieweck R, Kiebler MA, Popper B. mTOR and MAPK: From localized translation control to epilepsy. BMC Neuroscience. 2016;**17**(1):73

[123] Pires G, Leitner D, Drummond E, Kanshin E, Nayak S, Askenazi M, et al. Proteomic differences in the hippocampus and cortex of epilepsy brain tissue. Brain Communications. 2021;**3**(2):fcab021

[124] Fiore R, Rajman M, Schwale C, Bicker S, Antoniou A, Bruehl C, et al. MiR-134-dependent regulation of Pumilio-2 is necessary for homeostatic synaptic depression. The EMBO Journal. 2014;**33**(19):2231-2246

[125] Schratt GM, Tuebing F, Nigh EA, Kane CG, Sabatini ME, Kiebler M, et al. A brain-specific microRNA regulates dendritic spine development. Nature. 2006;**439**(7074):283-289

[126] Hwang JY, Kaneko N, Noh KM, Pontarelli F, Zukin RS. The gene silencing transcription factor REST represses miR-132 expression in hippocampal neurons destined to die. Journal of Molecular Biology. 2014; **426**(20):3454-3466

[127] Jimenez-Mateos EM, Bray I, Sanz-Rodriguez A, Engel T, McKiernan RC, Mouri G, et al. miRNA expression profile after status epilepticus and hippocampal neuroprotection by targeting miR-132. The American Journal of Pathology. 2011;**179**(5):2519-2532

[128] Jimenez-Mateos EM, Engel T, Merino-Serrais P, McKiernan RC, Tanaka K, Mouri G, et al. Silencing microRNA-134 produces neuroprotective and prolonged seizure-suppressive effects. Nature Medicine. 2012;**18**(7):1087-1094

[129] Reschke CR, Silva LFA, Norwood BA, Senthilkumar K, Morris G, Sanz-Rodriguez A, et al. Potent anti-seizure effects of locked nucleic acid antagomirs targeting miR-134 in multiple mouse and rat models of epilepsy. Molecular Therapy—Nucleic Acids. 2017;**6**:45-56

[130] Jimenez-Mateos EM, Engel T, Merino-Serrais P, Fernaud-Espinosa I, Rodriguez-Alvarez N, Reynolds J, et al. Antagomirs targeting microRNA-134 increase hippocampal pyramidal neuron spine volume in vivo and protect against pilocarpine-induced status epilepticus. Brain Structure & Function. 2015; **220**(4):2387-2399

[131] Gross C, Yao X, Engel T, Tiwari D, Xing L, Rowley S, et al. MicroRNA-mediated downregulation of the potassium channel Kv4.2 contributes to seizure onset. Cell Reports. 2016;**17**(1): 37-45

[132] Sakai A, Saitow F, Maruyama M, Miyake N, Miyake K, Shimada T, et al. MicroRNA cluster miR-17-92 regulates multiple functionally related voltage-gated potassium channels in chronic neuropathic pain. Nature Communications. 2017;**8**(1):16079

[133] Lippi G, Fernandes CC, Ewell LA, John D, Romoli B, Curia G, et al. MicroRNA-101 regulates multiple developmental programs to constrain excitation in adult neural networks. Neuron. 2016;**92**(6):1337-1351

[134] Rajman M, Metge F, Fiore R, Khudayberdiev S, Aksoy-Aksel A, Bicker S, et al. A microRNA-129-5p/Rbfox crosstalk coordinates homeostatic downscaling of excitatory synapses. The EMBO Journal. 2017;**36**(12):1770-1787

[135] Hogg MC, Raoof R, El Naggar H, Monsefi N, Delanty N, O'Brien DF, et al. Elevation of plasma tRNA fragments precedes seizures in human epilepsy. The Journal of Clinical Investigation. 2019;**129**(7):2946-2951

[136] Khoo SK, Petillo D, Kang UJ, Resau JH, Berryhill B, Linder J, et al. Plasma-based circulating MicroRNA biomarkers for Parkinson's disease. Journal of Parkinson's Disease. 2012;**2**(4):321-331

[137] Li N, Pan X, Zhang J, Ma A, Yang S, Ma J, et al. Plasma levels of miR-137 and miR-124 are associated with Parkinson's disease but not with Parkinson's disease with depression. Neurological Sciences. 2017;**38**(5):761-767

[138] Ma W, Li Y, Wang C, Xu F, Wang M, Liu Y. Serum miR-221 serves as a biomarker for Parkinson's disease. Cell Biochemistry and Function. 2016;**34**(7):511-515

[139] Dong H, Wang C, Lu S, Yu C, Huang L, Feng W, et al. A panel of four decreased serum microRNAs as a novel biomarker for early Parkinson's disease. Biomarkers. 2016;**21**(2):129-137

[140] Ding H, Huang Z, Chen M, Wang C, Chen X, Chen J, et al. Identification of a panel of five serum miRNAs as a biomarker for Parkinson's disease. Parkinsonism & Related Disorders. 2016;**22**:68-73

[141] Margis R, Margis R, Rieder CR. Identification of blood microRNAs associated to Parkinsonĭs disease. Journal of Biotechnology. 2011;**152**(3): 96-101

[142] Galimberti D, Villa C, Fenoglio C, Serpente M, Ghezzi L, Cioffi SM, et al. Circulating miRNAs as potential biomarkers in Alzheimer's disease. Journal of Alzheimer's Disease. 2014;**42**(4):1261-1267

[143] Tan L, Yu JT, Liu QY, Tan MS, Zhang W, Hu N, et al. Circulating miR-125b as a biomarker of Alzheimer's disease. Journal of the Neurological Sciences. 2014;**336**(1-2):52-56

[144] Kumar P, Dezso Z, MacKenzie C, Oestreicher J, Agoulnik S, Byrne M, et al. Circulating miRNA biomarkers for Alzheimer's disease. PLoS One. 2013;**8**(7):e69807

[145] Leidinger P, Backes C, Deutscher S, Schmitt K, Mueller SC, Frese K, et al. A blood based 12-miRNA signature of Alzheimer disease patients. Genome Biology. 2013;**14**(7):R78

[146] Cheng L, Doecke JD, Sharples RA, Villemagne VL, Fowler CJ, Rembach A, et al. Prognostic serum miRNA biomarkers associated with Alzheimer's disease shows concordance with neuropsychological and neuroimaging assessment. Molecular Psychiatry. 2015;**20**(10):1188-1196

[147] Bejleri J, Jirström E, Donovan P, Williams DJ, Pfeiffer S. Diagnostic and Prognostic Circulating MicroRNA in Acute Stroke: A Systematic and Bioinformatic Analysis of Current Evidence. J Stroke. 2021;**23**(2):162-182

[148] Tian C, Li Z, Yang Z, Huang Q, Liu J, Hong B. Plasma MicroRNA-16 Is a Biomarker for Diagnosis, Stratification, and Prognosis of Hyperacute Cerebral Infarction. PLoS One. 2016;**11**(11): e0166688

[149] Leung LY, Chan CP, Leung YK, Jiang HL, Abrigo JM, Wang de F, et al. Comparison of miR-124-3p and miR-16 for early diagnosis of hemorrhagic and ischemic stroke. Clinica Chimica Acta. 2014;**433**:139-144

[150] Jin F, Xing J. Circulating miR-126 and miR-130a levels correlate with lower disease risk, disease severity, and reduced inflammatory cytokine levels in acute ischemic stroke patients. Neurological Sciences. 2018;**39**(10): 1757-1765

[151] Jin F, Xing J. Circulating pro-angiogenic and anti-angiogenic microRNA expressions in patients with acute ischemic stroke and their association with disease severity. Neurological Sciences. 2017;**38**(11): 2015-2023

[152] Long G, Wang F, Li H, Yin Z, Sandip C, Lou Y, et al. Circulating miR-30a, miR-126 and let-7b as biomarker for ischemic stroke in humans. BMC Neurology. 2013;**13**:178

[153] Zhao B, Zhu Z, Hao J, Wan Z, Guo X. Decreased plasma miR-335 expression in patients with acute ischemic stroke and its association with calmodulin expression. The Journal of International Medical Research. 2016;**44**(6):1331-1338

[154] Wang MD, Wang Y, Xia YP, Dai JW, Gao L, Wang SQ, et al. High

serum MiR-130a levels are associated with severe perihematomal edema and predict adverse outcome in acute ICH. Molecular Neurobiology. 2016;**53**(2): 1310-1321

[155] Freischmidt A, Müller K, Ludolph AC, Weishaupt JH. Systemic dysregulation of TDP-43 binding microRNAs in amyotrophic lateral sclerosis. Acta Neuropathologica Communications. 2013;**1**:42

[156] Freischmidt A, Müller K, Zondler L, Weydt P, Mayer B, von Arnim CA, et al. Serum microRNAs in sporadic amyotrophic lateral sclerosis. Neurobiology of Aging. 2015;**36**(9): 2660.e15-2660.e20

[157] Waller R, Goodall EF, Milo M, Cooper-Knock J, Da Costa M, Hobson E, et al. Serum miRNAs miR-206, 143-3p and 374b-5p as potential biomarkers for amyotrophic lateral sclerosis (ALS). Neurobiology of Aging. 2017;**55**:123-131

[158] Wang J, Yu J-T, Tan L, Tian Y, Ma J, Tan C-C, et al. Genome-wide circulating microRNA expression profiling indicates biomarkers for epilepsy. Scientific Reports. 2015;**5**(1):9522

[159] Wang J, Tan L, Tan L, Tian Y, Ma J, Tan C-C, et al. Circulating microRNAs are promising novel biomarkers for drug-resistant epilepsy. Scientific Reports. 2015;**5**:10201

[160] Raoof R, Bauer S, El Naggar H, Connolly NMC, Brennan GP, Brindley E, et al. Dual-center, dual-platform microRNA profiling identifies potential plasma biomarkers of adult temporal lobe epilepsy. eBioMedicine. 2018;**38**:127-141

[161] Dammes N, Peer D. Paving the road for RNA therapeutics. Trends in Pharmacological Sciences. 2020;**41**(10): 755-775

[162] Judge AD, Bola G, Lee AC, MacLachlan I. Design of noninflammatory synthetic siRNA mediating potent gene silencing in vivo. Molecular Therapy. 2006;**13**(3):494-505

[163] Sioud M. Single-stranded small interfering RNA are more immunostimulatory than their double-stranded counterparts: A central role for 2′-hydroxyl uridines in immune responses. European Journal of Immunology. 2006;**36**(5):1222-1230

[164] Cirak S, Arechavala-Gomeza V, Guglieri M, Feng L, Torelli S, Anthony K, et al. Exon skipping and dystrophin restoration in patients with Duchenne muscular dystrophy after systemic phosphorodiamidate morpholino oligomer treatment: An open-label, phase 2, dose-escalation study. Lancet. 2011;**378**(9791):595-605

[165] Winkle M, El-Daly SM, Fabbri M, Calin GA. Noncoding RNA therapeutics—Challenges and potential solutions. Nature Reviews Drug Discovery. 2021;**20**(8):629-651

[166] Jin HY, Gonzalez-Martin A, Miletic AV, Lai M, Knight S, Sabouri-Ghomi M, et al. Transfection of microRNA mimics should be used with caution. Frontiers in Genetics. 2015;**6**:340

[167] Bonneau E, Neveu B, Kostantin E, Tsongalis GJ, De Guire V. How close are miRNAs from clinical practice? A perspective on the diagnostic and therapeutic market. EJIFCC. 2019; **30**(2):114-127